Study Guide

for

Understanding Nursing Research

Third Edition

Study Guide
for
Understanding Nursing Research

Third Edition

NANCY BURNS, PhD, RN, FAAN

Jenkins Garrett Professor
School of Nursing
The University of Texas at Arlington
Arlington, Texas

SUSAN K. GROVE, PhD, RN, ANP, GNP, APRN, BC

Professor of Nursing
Assistant Dean, Graduate Nursing Program
School of Nursing
The University of Texas at Arlington
Arlington, Texas

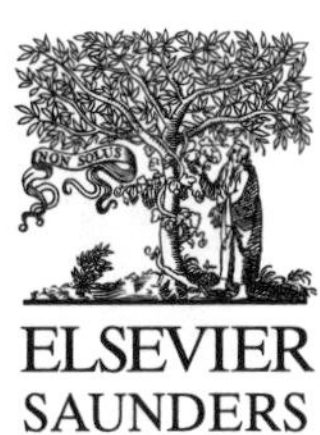

ELSEVIER
SAUNDERS

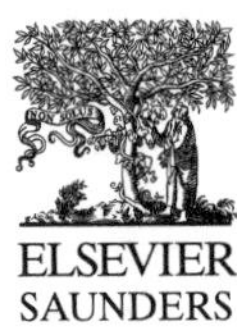

ELSEVIER
SAUNDERS

The Curtis Center
Independence Square West
Philadelphia, Pennsylvania 19106-3399

Study Guide for
Understanding Nursing Research, Third edition

ISBN 0-7216-0012-3

Vice President and Publishing Director, Nursing: Sally Schrefer
Executive Publisher: Barbara Nelson Cullen
Developmental Editor: Victoria Bruno
Project Manager: Gayle May
Designer: Wordbench
Cover Art: Julia Dummitt

WB/FF

Printed in the United States of America

Last digit is the print number: 9 8 7 6 5 4 3 2

Preface

The amount of knowledge generated through research is rapidly escalating in nursing. This empirical knowledge is critical for developing an evidence-based practice in nursing that is both high-quality and cost-effective for patients, families, providers, and health care agencies. As a baccalaureate-prepared nurse, you will be encouraged to read and use research findings to develop protocols, algorithms, and policies for practice. We will also provide you direction for using national developed guidelines in your practice. We recognize that learning research terminology and reading and critiquing research reports are complex and sometimes overwhelming activities. Thus, we have developed this Study Guide to assist you in clarifying, comprehending, analyzing, synthesizing, and applying the content presented in your textbook, *Understanding Nursing Research* (3rd edition). This edition of the Study Guide is organized according to the steps of the research process and includes exercises that address the revised content on literature review, sampling, and statistics.

Your Study Guide is organized into 13 chapters, which are consistent with the chapters of your textbook. Each chapter of your study guide presents you with learning exercises that require various levels of critical thinking skills. These exercises are organized using the following headings: Relevant Terms, Key Ideas, Making Connections, Puzzles, Exercises in Critique, and Going Beyond. In some exercises, you will define relevant terms or identify key ideas. In other exercises, you will demonstrate comprehension of the research process by connecting one idea to another. Some exercises are puzzles that will make learning research fun. In the most complex exercises, you will apply your new research knowledge by conducting critiques of published studies.

After completing the exercises for each chapter, you will be able to review the answers in Appendix A and assess your understanding of the content. Based on your correct and incorrect responses, you will be able to focus your study to improve your knowledge of each chapter's content.

Since your learning is enhanced by exposure to a variety of visual exercises, we have included over 300 online multiple-choice questions to accompany the Study Guide. You can locate these questions on the Evolve Burns and Grove Student Learning Resources website at http://evolve.elsevier.com/Burns/understanding. You'll also want to check out the WebLinks and the Learning Resources to accompany the text—also located on Evolve. The WebLinks provide links to various related websites for each chapter. The Learning Resources are "open-book quizzes" including crossword puzzles, fill-in-the-blank questions, matching questions, and multiple-choice questions for each chapter.

Completing the exercises in the student study guide and online can provide you with a background for analyzing and synthesizing the findings from research reports for application in practice.

Introduction

This Study Guide was developed to accompany the textbook *Understanding Nursing Research*, 3rd edition. The exercises in this guide were designed to assist you in comprehending the content in your textbook, conducting critiques of nursing studies, and using research findings in practice. You need to read each chapter in your text before completing the chapters in this guide. Scan the entire chapter to get an overall view of the content. Then reread the chapter with the intent of increasing your comprehension of each section. As you examine each section, pay careful attention to the terms that are defined. If the meaning of a term is not clear to you, look up its definition in the glossary at the back of the book or in a dictionary. Highlight key ideas in each section. Examine tables and figures as they are referred to in the text. Mark sections you do not feel you sufficiently understand. Jot down questions to ask your instructor in class or privately.

After carefully reading a chapter in the text, use the Study Guide and online questions and exercises to further enhance your understanding of the research process. Each chapter in the Study Guide corresponds to its related chapter in your textbook. There are six main sections to each Study Guide chapter: Relevant Terms, Key Ideas, Making Connections, Puzzles, Exercises in Critique, and Going Beyond.

Relevant Terms

Relevant terms have been identified for each chapter to assist you in becoming familiar with essential terminology for understanding the research process. Knowing these terms before you attend a class lecture on the content will give you an edge in grasping the lecture content and doing well on course exams. As you read the text, do not skip over terms in the chapter that are unfamiliar to you. Get in the habit of marking unfamiliar words as you read and looking up their definitions in the glossary at the end of the text.

Key Ideas

This section of the Study Guide identifies important information in each chapter for you. The fill-in-the-blank questions include both short and long answer formats and will assist you in identifying essential chapter content that you might have missed. You may need to refer to specific sections of the text to complete some of the questions.

Making Connections

The Making Connections exercises promote linking ideas to facilitate the comprehending, analyzing, and synthesizing of content related to the research process. Matching questions are frequently used to assist you in performing these critical thinking skills.

Puzzles

The Puzzles section is designed for having fun while learning the research process. The Crossword Puzzles were developed to help you increase your familiarity with the terms used in the chapter. The Word Scrambles contain important ideas expressed in the chapter, but the letters in each word have been scrambled. For example, "study" might be scrambled to read "tysud." You will need to unscramble the words to get the message. The Secret Messages contain other important ideas expressed in the chapter. To decipher these messages, you must identify the code used and decode the message. For example, one secret message might have been coded by moving each letter of the alphabet down three letters. In this case, A = D, B = E, C = F, etc. Once you identify a few letters, you have clues you can use to guess at other letters in words. You may find it easier to start with the short words. Also, remember that the most commonly used letter in our language is *e*.

Exercises in Critique

Critique exercises are provided to give you experiences in critiquing published studies. In some cases, brief quotes are provided with questions addressing information specific to the chapter content. The critique exercises focus on the three published studies that are provided in Appendix B of this Study Guide. On completing the Study Guide, you can incorporate the critique information you have learned to perform an overall critique of these three studies. In addition, you can take the knowledge you have learned and apply it in the critique of other published studies.

Going Beyond

Exercises have been included that provide suggestions for further study. You might use these activities to test your new knowledge. If the content of a particular chapter interests you, this section might direct you in learning more about that step of the research process.

Answers

The answers to all Study Guide questions are provided in Appendix A in the back of the Study Guide. However, we recommend that you not refer to these answers except to check your own responses to the questions. You will learn more by reading the textbook and searching for the answers on your own.

Published Studies

Reprints of three published studies are provided in Appendix B. These studies are referred to in many of the study questions throughout the Study Guide.

Contents

chapter 1 Discovering Nursing Research

INTRODUCTION

You need to read Chapter 1 and then complete the following exercises. These exercises will assist you in learning relevant terms and identifying the types of research conducted in nursing. The answers to these exercises are in Appendix A under Chapter 1.

RELEVANT TERMS

Directions: Match each term below with its correct definition.

a. Authority
b. Deductive reasoning
c. Explanation
d. Inductive reasoning
e. Intuition
f. Knowledge
g. Nursing research
h. Outcomes research
i. Personal experience
j. Prediction
k. Qualitative research
l. Quantitative research
m. Reasoning
n. Research
o. Scientific methods
p. Trial and error

Definitions

_____ 1. Information acquired in a variety of ways that is expected to be an accurate reflection of reality.

_____ 2. Scientific process that validates and refines existing knowledge and generates new knowledge that directly and indirectly influences nursing practice.

_____ 3. Person with expertise and power who is able to influence the opinion of others.

_____ 4. Reasoning from the specific to the general.

_____ 5. Gaining knowledge by being personally involved in an event, situation, or circumstance.

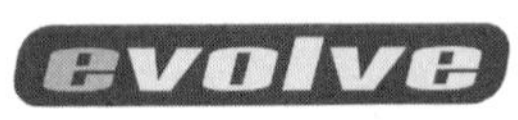

Be sure to check out the free exercises on-line at http://evolve.elsevier.com/Burns/understanding

_____ 6. Formal, objective, systematic research process to describe, test relationships, or examine cause-and-effect interactions among variables.

_____ 7. Reasoning from the general to the specific or from a general premise to a particular situation.

_____ 8. Procedures that scientists have used, currently use, or may use in the future to pursue knowledge.

_____ 9. Insight or understanding of a situation or event as a whole that usually cannot be logically explained.

_____ 10. Diligent, systematic inquiry to validate and refine existing knowledge and generate new knowledge.

_____ 11. Systematic, subjective research approach used to describe life experiences and give them meaning.

_____ 12. Knowledge generated from research that clarifies relationships among variables and identifies the reasons why certain events occur.

_____ 13. An important scientific methodology that was developed to examine the end results of patient care.

_____ 14. Type of thinking that involves processing and organizing ideas in order to reach conclusions.

_____ 15. Knowledge generated from research that enables one to estimate the probability of a specific outcome in a given situation.

_____ 16. An approach with unknown outcomes that is used in a situation of uncertainty in which other sources of knowledge are unavailable. Often unique, individual patient situations require use of this approach.

KEY IDEAS

Directions: The knowledge generated through research is essential to provide a scientific basis for **description**, **explanation**, **prediction**, and **control** of nursing practice. Write a definition and provide an example of these four terms.

1. Description: ____________________

____

____

Example: ____________________

2. Explanation: ____________________

____

____

Example: ____________________

3. Prediction: ____

____

____

Example: ____

4. Control: ____

____

____

Example: ____

Historical Events Influencing Nursing Research

Directions: Fill in the blanks in this section with the appropriate word(s) or numbers.

1. ______________________ is considered the first nurse researcher.
2. The journal *Nursing Research* was first published in __________.
3. The American Nurses Association (ANA) Commission on Nursing Research established the ____ in 1972.
4. Many national and international ______________ conferences have been sponsored by Sigma Theta Tau, the international honor society for nursing since 1970.
5. The nursing research journal first published in 1978 is ______________________ ______________________.
6. The research journal first published in 1979 is ______________________ ______________________.
7. Identify three other research journals that were first published in 1987 or 1988.
   a. ____
   b. ____
   c. ____
8. ____ was the project directed by Horsley to promote the use of research findings in practice, and the project results were published in 1982–1983.

9. The *Annual Review of Nursing Research* includes ______________________________
____.

10. The National Center for Nursing Research (NCNR) was established in ____________ by the National Institutes for Health.

11. The NCNR is now called the ____.

12. The purpose of the National Institute for Nursing Research (NINR) is ________________________________, ______________________________, and ______________________________________ regarding basic and clinical nursing research.

13. Identify the mission of the NINR for the 21st century.
____
____
____
____

14. The focus of nursing research in the 1980s and 1990s was the conduct of ____________________ research.

15. ____ was established in 1989 to facilitate the conduct of outcomes research and the communication of the findings to health care practitioners.

16. The conduct of numerous high-quality studies is essential for the development of a(n) ________________________ knowledge base for nursing practice.

17. The Agency for Health Care Policy and Research (AHCPR) was renamed in 1999 to the ____.
This agency is playing a major role in the development of evidence-based guidelines for use in practice.

18. Evidence-based practice is the focus of the 21st century and involves the synthesis of knowledge from quantitative, qualitative, and outcomes research in:
a. ____
b. ____
c. ____

19. The Department of Health and Human Services (DHHS) increased the visibility of and identified priorities for health promotion research by publishing

    ____.

20. The type of research that is focused on quality and cost-effectiveness of health care, which increased in the 1900s and will continue to expand in the 21st century, is ______________________________.

Acquiring Knowledge in Nursing

Directions: Fill in the blanks with the appropriate responses.

1. List seven ways of acquiring knowledge in nursing and provide an example of each.
   a. ______________________________
   b. ______________________________
   c. ______________________________
   d. ______________________________
   e. ______________________________
   f. ______________________________
   g. ______________________________
2. Benner's 1984 book, *From Novice to Expert: Excellence and Power in Clinical Practice,* describes the importance of ______________________________ in acquiring nursing knowledge.
3. Identify Benner's five levels of experience in the development of clinical knowledge and expertise.
   a. ______________________________
   b. ______________________________
   c. ______________________________
   d. ______________________________
   e. ______________________________
4. Nursing has ____________________ knowledge from other disciplines such as medicine, psychology, and sociology.

5. ______________________ knowledge provides an evidence base for description, explanation, prediction, and control of nursing practice.
6. A "gut feeling" or "hunch" is an example of ____________________________, which nurses have found useful in identifying serious patients' problems.
7. ________________________ are knowledge based on customs and past trends, such as providing hospitalized patients a bath every morning.
8. New graduates sometimes enter internships provided by clinical agencies and are guided, supported, and educated by experienced nurses. This is an example of a ____.
9. In the internship, new graduates are encouraged to ___________________________ or imitate the behaviors of expert nurses.
10. Two types of logical reasoning are ______________________________ and ______________________________.
11. What type of reasoning is used in the following example? ______________________
    Human beings experience pain.
    Babies are human beings.
    Therefore, babies experience pain.
12. The types of research that are essential for the generation of knowledge for nursing practice are ____________________________, ____________________________, and __________________________________.
13. What type of research is conducted to examine the cost-effectiveness of health care? ____________________________________

14. Identify five interventions that you use frequently in your nursing practice. Next to each intervention, identify the knowledge base for that intervention.

Intervention	Knowledge Base
a.	
b.	
c.	
d.	
e.	

15. What type of knowledge is the basis for the majority of your interventions in clinical practice?

16. Identify four important outcomes that might be examined with outcomes research.
    a. ______________________________
    b. ______________________________
    c. ______________________________
    d. ______________________________

MAKING CONNECTIONS

Directions: Match the following research methods with the specific types of research.

Types of Research Methods

a. Qualitative research method
b. Quantitative research method

Types of Research

_____ 1. Correlational research
_____ 2. Descriptive research
_____ 3. Ethnographic research
_____ 4. Experimental research
_____ 5. Grounded theory research
_____ 6. Historical research
_____ 7. Phenomenological research
_____ 8. Quasi-experimental research

Directions: Match the levels of nurses' educational preparation with the research activities that each group of nurses is primarily responsible for according to the guidelines of the American Nurses Association (ANA).

Nurses' Educational Preparation

a. Associate degree
b. Baccalaureate degree
c. Master's degree
d. Doctoral degree (PhD or DNS)
e. Postdoctorate

Research Activities

_____ 1. Uses research findings in practice with supervision
_____ 2. Develops and coordinates funded research programs
_____ 3. Critiques studies
_____ 4. Develops nursing knowledge through research and theory development
_____ 5. Uses research findings in practice
_____ 6. Collaborates in conducting research projects
_____ 7. Conducts independent research projects

PUZZLES

Word Scramble

Qtiutaantive, aliqutaivte, and tousemoc sereacrh era esenstial to evledpo viednaec-sabde singnur tprcacie.

Searerch nowkdegle si deende to trconol tcosuome in urinngs actripce.

EXERCISES IN CRITIQUE

Directions: Locate the research articles (listed below) in Appendix B. Review the titles, abstracts, introductions, and methodology of these three articles. Identify the type of research conducted in each study. Remember, some studies combine both quantitative and qualitative research methods in conducting a study.

Research Methods

a. Outcomes research method
b. Qualitative research method
c. Quantitative research method

_____ 1. Carey, Nicholson, and Fox (2002) study
_____ 2. Lewis, Nichols, Mackey, Fadol, Sloane, Villagomez, and Liehr (1997) study
_____ 3. Bruce and Grove (1994) study

Researchers' Credentials

Directions: Review the educational and clinical credentials of the authors of the three research articles in Appendix B.

1. Discuss whether or not Carey et al. (2002) had the educational and clinical preparation to conduct their study.

2. Discuss whether or not Lewis et al. (1997) had the educational and clinical preparation to conduct their study.

3. Discuss whether or not Bruce and Grove (1994) had the educational and clinical preparation to conduct their study.

GOING BEYOND

1. Locate the most recent copy of one of these journals: *Applied Nursing Research* or *Nursing Research*. Identify the research method (qualitative, quantitative, or outcomes) used in each study in the journal. Provide a rationale for your answer. Ask your instructor to verify your answers.

2. Find a faculty member who is conducting research. Ask if you can participate in the collection of data for this project. Could this faculty member be a mentor to you in promoting your understanding of quantitative, qualitative, and outcomes research?

chapter 2 Introduction to the Quantitative Research Process

INTRODUCTION

You need to read Chapter 2 and then complete the following exercises. These exercises will assist you in learning the steps of the quantitative research process, identifying the different types of quantitative research (descriptive, correlational, quasi-experimental, and experimental), and reading research reports. The answers for the following exercises are in Appendix A under Chapter 2.

RELEVANT TERMS

Directions: Match each term below with its correct definition.

a. Abstract
b. Applied research
c. Assumption
d. Basic research
e. Control
f. Design
g. Framework
h. Generalization
i. Methodological limitations
j. Methods section of a research report
k. Nursing process
l. Pilot study
m. Problem-solving process
n. Quantitative research process
o. Reading research reports
p. Research report
q. Rigor
r. Sampling
s. Setting
t. Theoretical limitations

Definitions

_____ 1. Formal, objective, systematic process to describe, test relationships, and examine cause-and-effect interactions among variables.

_____ 2. Location for conducting research that can be natural, partially controlled, or highly controlled.

_____ 3. Scientific investigations conducted to generate knowledge that will directly influence clinical practice.

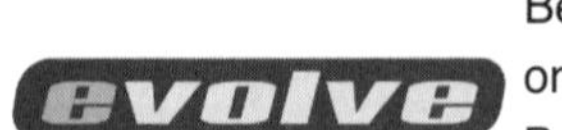

Be sure to check out the free exercises on-line at http://evolve.elsevier.com/Burns/understanding

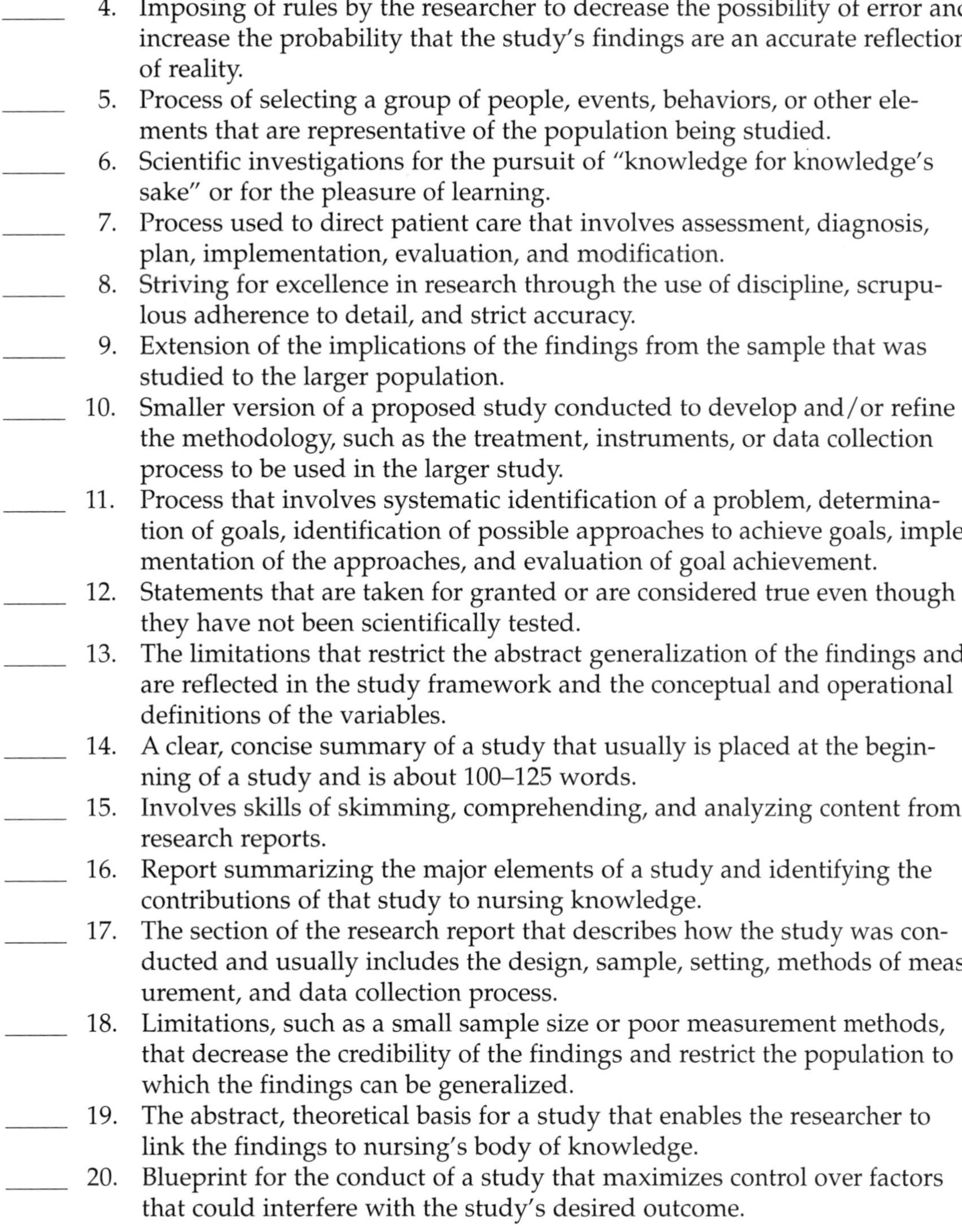

_____ 4. Imposing of rules by the researcher to decrease the possibility of error and increase the probability that the study's findings are an accurate reflection of reality.

_____ 5. Process of selecting a group of people, events, behaviors, or other elements that are representative of the population being studied.

_____ 6. Scientific investigations for the pursuit of "knowledge for knowledge's sake" or for the pleasure of learning.

_____ 7. Process used to direct patient care that involves assessment, diagnosis, plan, implementation, evaluation, and modification.

_____ 8. Striving for excellence in research through the use of discipline, scrupulous adherence to detail, and strict accuracy.

_____ 9. Extension of the implications of the findings from the sample that was studied to the larger population.

_____ 10. Smaller version of a proposed study conducted to develop and/or refine the methodology, such as the treatment, instruments, or data collection process to be used in the larger study.

_____ 11. Process that involves systematic identification of a problem, determination of goals, identification of possible approaches to achieve goals, implementation of the approaches, and evaluation of goal achievement.

_____ 12. Statements that are taken for granted or are considered true even though they have not been scientifically tested.

_____ 13. The limitations that restrict the abstract generalization of the findings and are reflected in the study framework and the conceptual and operational definitions of the variables.

_____ 14. A clear, concise summary of a study that usually is placed at the beginning of a study and is about 100–125 words.

_____ 15. Involves skills of skimming, comprehending, and analyzing content from research reports.

_____ 16. Report summarizing the major elements of a study and identifying the contributions of that study to nursing knowledge.

_____ 17. The section of the research report that describes how the study was conducted and usually includes the design, sample, setting, methods of measurement, and data collection process.

_____ 18. Limitations, such as a small sample size or poor measurement methods, that decrease the credibility of the findings and restrict the population to which the findings can be generalized.

_____ 19. The abstract, theoretical basis for a study that enables the researcher to link the findings to nursing's body of knowledge.

_____ 20. Blueprint for the conduct of a study that maximizes control over factors that could interfere with the study's desired outcome.

KEY IDEAS

Control in Quantitative Research

Directions: Fill in the blanks with the appropriate word(s).

1. An experimental study is conducted in a ______________________________ setting.
2. Extraneous variables need to be controlled in ______________________________ and ____ types of quantitative research to ensure that the findings are an accurate reflection of reality.
3. ______________________________ or ______________________________ studies are usually uncontrolled by the researcher and conducted in natural settings.
4. ___________________________________ studies require random selection of the sample.
5. Frequently a ______________________________ sampling method is used in descriptive and correlational studies. However, a ______________________________ sampling method might also be used.
6. Subjects' home is an example of a ______________________________ setting.
7. Laboratories or research centers are examples of ______________________________ settings.
8. Researcher control is greatest in what type of quantitative research?

    ____
9. Hospital units are ____ settings that allow the researcher to control some of the extraneous variables.
10. ___________________________________ research is conducted to determine the effect of a treatment but often involves less control than experimental research.

Steps of the Research Process

Directions: Fill in the blanks with the appropriate word(s).

1. The research process is similar to the ____________________________ and the _____________________ processes.

2. The nursing diagnosis step of the nursing process is similar to the ____________________ and ____________________________________ of the research process.
3. The plan of the nursing process is similar to the ______________________________ step of the research process.
4. The evaluation and modification steps of the nursing process are similar to the ________________________________ and ____________________________ steps of the problem-solving process. However, the last steps of the research process of, ________________________________, ____________________________________, and ____________________________________ are quite different.
5. List the steps of the quantitative research process in their order of occurrence.
   Step 1 ____
   Step 2 ____
   Step 3 ____
   Step 4 ____
   Step 5 ____
   Step 6 ____
   Step 7 ____
   Step 8 ____
   Step 9 ____
   Step 10 ____
   Step 11 ____
   Step 12 ____
   Step 13 ____
6. Assumptions are ____
   ____
   ____.
7. Identify four common assumptions on which nursing studies have been based.
   a. ____
   b. ____
   c. ____
   d. ____

8. The two types of limitations that might exist in a study are ______________________ and ______________________.
9. Identify five possible examples of limitations that you might find in published studies.
   a. ______________________
   b. ______________________
   c. ______________________
   d. ______________________
   e. ______________________
10. A pilot study is ______________________
    ______________________.
11. Identify five reasons for conducting a pilot study.
    a. ______________________
    b. ______________________
    c. ______________________
    d. ______________________
    e. ______________________

Reading Research Reports

1. The most common sources for nursing research reports are professional journals. Identify three nursing research journals.
   a. ______________________
   b. ______________________
   c. ______________________
2. Identify three clinical journals in which research reports compose 50% or more of the journal content.
   a. ______________________
   b. ______________________
   c. ______________________
3. Identify the four major sections of a research report.
   a. ______________________ c. ______________________
   b. ______________________ d. ______________________

4. The methods section of a research report describes how a study was conducted and usually includes:

   a. ______________________ d. ______________________

   b. ______________________ e. ______________________

   c. ______________________

5. The discussion section ties the other sections of the research report together and gives them meaning. This section includes:

   a. ____

   b. ____

   c. ____

   d. ____

   e. ____

6. The problem and purpose are often identified in what section of a research report?

   ____

7. The reference list at the end of the article includes all the ____________________ and ____________________ that provide a basis for this study and are cited in the article.

8. Reading a research report involves ________________________, ________________________, and ________________________ the content of the report.

9. In reading a research report, the ________________________ step involves identifying the steps of the research process.

10. In reading a research report, ________________________ involves determining the value of the report's content by determining the quality and completeness of the steps of the research process and examining logical links among these steps.

MAKING CONNECTIONS

Types of Quantitative Research

Directions: Match the type of quantitative research listed below with the examples of study titles.

a. Descriptive research
b. Correlational research
c. Quasi-experimental research
d. Experimental research

_____ 1. Determining the effect of a relaxation technique on patients' postoperative pain and anxiety level.
_____ 2. Identifying the incidence of HIV in adolescents and young adults.
_____ 3. Examining the relationships among age, gender, knowledge of AIDS, and use of condoms in college students.
_____ 4. Describing the coping strategies of chronically ill men and women.
_____ 5. Determining the effects of position on sacral and heel pressures in hospitalized elderly.
_____ 6. Determining the effect of impaired physical mobility on skeletal muscle atrophy in laboratory rats.
_____ 7. Identifying current nursing practice for male and female nurses.
_____ 8. Examining the relationship among intensive care unit (ICU) stress, anxiety, and recovery rate for patients following cardiac surgery.
_____ 9. Examining the effects of a preadmission self-instruction program on patients' postoperative activity level, anxiety level, pain perception, length of hospital stay, and time to return to work.
_____ 10. Examining the effects of thermal applications on the abdominal temperature of laboratory dogs.
_____ 11. Examining the relationships among hardiness, depression, and coping in institutionalized elderly.
_____ 12. Determining the incidence of drug abuse in registered nurses in community and hospital settings.
_____ 13. Examining the effect of warm and cold applications on the resolution of IV infiltrations in hospitalized patients.
_____ 14. Determining the stress levels and desired support of family caregivers of elderly with Alzheimer's disease.
_____ 15. Examining the effectiveness of a breast cancer screening program for women residing in rural areas.
_____ 16. Comparing the age and coping skills of mothers pregnant with their first child in three ethnic groups (Caucasian, African American, and Hispanic).

_____ 17. Using age, nutritional intake, mobility level, weight, level of cognitive function, and serum albumin to predict the risk for pressure ulcers in hospitalized patients on a medical-surgical unit.

_____ 18. Describing the severity of fatigue and anxiety in individuals with chronic obstructive pulmonary disease.

_____ 19. Comparing and contrasting the health promotion and illness prevention behaviors of African American and Caucasian older adults.

_____ 20. Examining the relationships among the lipid values, blood pressure, weight, and stress levels of adolescents.

PUZZLES

Word Scramble

1. Taquntiatiev sereacrh thodmes duclein cridpseitve, rrelacotiaonl, saiqu-perexienmtal, dna eperxmiealnt udiests.

2. Gorir dan rotconl ear pormtinta ni utitavieqtan chrearse.

Crossword Puzzle

Directions: Complete the crossword puzzle below. Note that if the answer is more than one word, there are no blank spaces left between the words.

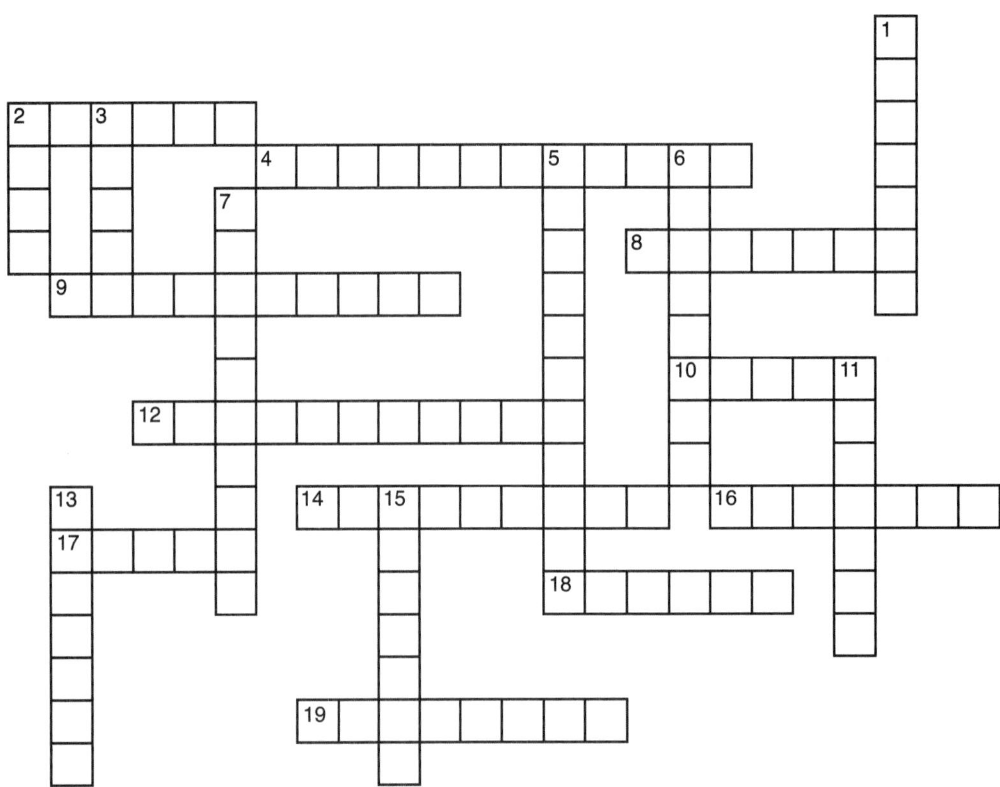

ACROSS

2. Study blueprint.
4. Research method.
8. Nursing concern.
9. Null ____.
10. Type of research that seeks knowledge for knowledge's sake.
12. _____ of dependent variables in research.
14. Crisis theory could be a study ____.
16. Location of research.
17. Strict adherence to research plan.
18. Subjects comprise this.
19. Directs a study.

DOWN

1. Research finding.
2. What is collected in a study?
3. Research project.
5. Known truths.
6. Study treatment is an independent _________.
7. What is reviewed prior to conducting a study?
11. Researchers ______ extraneous variables.
13. Nursing ______ to direct nursing care.
15. Practice-related studies are _____ research.

EXERCISES IN CRITIQUE

Directions: Read the research articles in Appendix B and answer the following questions.

Type of Quantitative Research

Identify the type of quantitative research conducted in each study.

a. Descriptive research
b. Correlational research
c. Quasi-experimental research
d. Experimental research

_____ 1. "Maternal Factors Related to Parenting Young Children with Congenital Heart Disease" (Carey, Nicholson, & Fox, 2002).
_____ 2. "The Effect of Turning and Backrub on Mixed Venous Oxygen Saturation in Critically Ill Patients" (Lewis, Nichols, Mackey, Fadol, Sloane, Villagomez, & Liehr, 1997).
_____ 3. "The Effect of a Coronary Artery Risk Evaluation Program on Serum Lipid Values and Cardiovascular Risk Levels" (Bruce & Grove, 1994).

Type of Setting

Identify the type of setting for each study.

a. Natural setting
b. Partially controlled setting
c. Highly controlled setting

_____ 4. Carey et al. (2002) study
_____ 5. Lewis et al. (1997) study
_____ 6. Bruce and Grove (1994) study

Type of Research Conducted (Applied or Basic)

Indicate the type of nursing research conducted in each study.

a. Applied nursing research
b. Basic nursing research

_____ 7. Carey et al. (2002) study
_____ 8. Lewis et al. (1997) study
_____ 9. Bruce and Grove (1994) study

chapter 3 Research Problems, Purposes, and Hypotheses

INTRODUCTION

You need to read Chapter 3 and then complete the following exercises. These exercises will assist you in critiquing problems, purposes, objectives, questions, hypotheses, and variables in published studies. The answers to these exercises are in Appendix A under Chapter 3.

RELEVANT TERMS

Directions: Match each term below with its correct definition.

a. Conceptual definition of variable
b. Demographic variable
c. Dependent variable
d. Hypothesis
e. Independent variable
f. Landmark study
g. Operational definition of variable
h. Research problem
i. Research purpose
j. Research question
k. Research topic

Definitions

_____ 1. Major, significant study generating knowledge that influences a discipline and sometimes society.
_____ 2. Clear, concise statement of the specific goal or aim of the study that is generated from the problem.
_____ 3. Area of concern or gap in the knowledge base that is needed for practice and requires study.
_____ 4. Description of how variables will be measured or manipulated in a study.
_____ 5. Concise interrogative statement developed to direct a study; focuses on description of variables, examination of relationships among variables, and determination of differences between two or more groups.
_____ 6. Concept or broad problem area that provides the basis for generating numerous research problems.

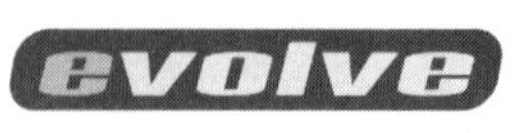

Be sure to check out the free exercises on-line at http://evolve.elsevier.com/Burns/understanding

_____ 7. The treatment or experimental activity that is manipulated or varied by the researcher to create an effect on the dependent variable.

_____ 8. Formal statement of the expected relationship or expected outcome between two or more variables in a specified population.

_____ 9. Definition that provides a variable or concept with connotative (abstract, comprehensive, theoretical) meaning; established through concept analysis, concept derivation, or concept synthesis.

_____ 10. The response, behavior, or outcome that is predicted or explained in research; changes in this variable are presumed to be caused by the independent variable.

_____ 11. Characteristics or attributes of subjects that are collected to describe the sample.

Types of Hypotheses

Directions: Match each type of hypothesis with the correct definition.

a. Associative hypothesis
b. Causal hypothesis
c. Complex hypothesis
d. Directional hypothesis
e. Nondirectional hypothesis
f. Null hypothesis
g. Research hypothesis
h. Simple hypothesis

Definitions

_____ 1. Hypothesis stating the relationship (associative or causal) between two variables.

_____ 2. Alternative hypothesis to the null hypothesis; states that a relationship exists between two or more variables.

_____ 3. Hypothesis stating a relationship between two variables in which one variable (independent variable) is thought to cause or determine the presence of the other variable (dependent variable).

_____ 4. Hypothesis stating that a relationship exists but does not predict the exact nature of the relationship.

_____ 5. Hypothesis predicting the relationships (associative or causal) among three or more variables.

_____ 6. Hypothesis stating a relationship in which variables or concepts that occur or exist together in the real world are identified; thus, when one variable changes, the other variable changes.

_____ 7. Hypothesis stating the specific nature of the interaction or relationship between two or more variables.

_____ 8. Hypothesis stating no relationship exists between the variables being studied.

Variables and Relevant Terms

Directions: Match these terms about variables with the appropriate example.

a. Conceptual definition
b. Demographic variable
c. Dependent variable
d. Extraneous variable
e. Independent variable
f. Operational definition

Definitions

_____ 1. Pain is a physiologic and psychological response to a stimulus that occurs whenever and to the degree that a patient says it does. This is an example of what type of definition?

_____ 2. Variables that exist in all studies and can affect the measurement of study variables and the relationships among these variables, such as changes in the environment, interaction with other people, or the health status of a patient.

_____ 3. The patients' pain will be measured with a visual analog scale and the Perception of Pain Likert Scale. This is an example of what type of definition?

_____ 4. The variables of heart rate, blood pressure, and respiratory rate that are measured after the completion of an exercise program.

_____ 5. Treatment of ambulating a patient every 2 hours.

_____ 6. Variables such as age, gender, and ethnic origin measured to describe the sample.

KEY IDEAS

Research Problem and Purpose

Directions: Fill in the blanks with the correct responses.

1. A clearly stated research purpose includes (a) ______________________________,
   (b) ______________________________,
   and usually the (c) ______________________________.
2. Research problems and purposes are significant if they have the potential to generate and refine relevant knowledge that:
   a. ______________________________
   b. ______________________________
   c. ______________________________
   d. ______________________________

3. Identify two organizations or agencies that have developed lists of research priorities relevant to nursing.
   a. ____________________
   b. ____________________
4. The feasibility of a research problem and purpose is determined by examining the following:
   a. ____________________
   b. ____________________
   c. ____________________
   d. ____________________
5. Two ways to determine researcher expertise is by examining the ____________ preparation and ____________ experience of the researchers.
6. ____________, ____________, and ____________ evolve from the study purpose and provide direction for the remaining steps of the research process.

EXERCISES IN CRITIQUE

Carey et al. Study

Directions: Review the Carey et al. (2002) article in Appendix B and answer the following questions.

1. State the problem of this study.

2. State the purpose of this study.

3. Are the problem and the purpose significant? Provide a rationale.

4. Does the purpose identify the variables, population, and setting for this study?

   a. Identify the variables.

   b. Identify the population.

   c. Identify the setting.

5. Are the problem and purpose feasible for the researchers to study? Provide a rationale.

Lewis et al. Study

Directions: Review the Lewis et al. (1997) article in Appendix B and answer the following questions.

1. State the problem of this study.

2. State the purpose of this study.

3. Are the problem and the purpose significant? Provide a rationale.

4. Does the purpose identify the variables, population, and setting for this study?

   a. Identify the variables.

   b. Identify the population.

   c. Identify the setting.

5. Are the problem and purpose feasible for the researchers to study? Provide a rationale.

Bruce and Grove Study

Directions: Review the Bruce and Grove (1994) article in Appendix B and answer the following questions.

1. State the problem of this study.

2. State the purpose of this study.

3. Are the problem and the purpose significant? Provide a rationale.

4. Does the purpose identify the variables, population, and setting for this study?

   a. Identify the variables.

   b. Identify the population.

   c. Identify the setting.

5. Are the problem and purpose feasible for the researchers to study? Provide a rationale.

MAKING CONNECTIONS

Objectives, Questions, and Hypotheses

Directions: Ten example hypotheses are listed below and on the next page. Identify each hypothesis using the terms listed below. Four terms are needed to identify each hypothesis. The correct answer for hypothesis #1 is provided as an example.

a. Associative hypothesis
b. Causal hypothesis
c. Complex hypothesis
d. Directional hypothesis
e. Nondirectional hypothesis
f. Null hypothesis
g. Research hypothesis
h. Simple hypothesis

__b, c, d, g__ 1. Relaxation therapy is more effective than standard care in decreasing pain perception and use of pain medications in adults with chronic arthritic pain.

_______________ 2. Age, family support, and health status are related to the self-care abilities of nursing home residents.

_______________ 3. Heparinized saline is no more effective than normal saline in maintaining the patency and comfort of a heparin lock.

_______________ 4. Poor health status is related to decreasing self-care abilities in institutionalized elderly.

_______________ 5. Low-back massage is more effective in decreasing perception of low-back pain than no massage in patients with chronic low-back pain.

_______________ 6. Healthy adults involved in a diet and exercise program have lower low-density lipoprotein (LDL), higher high-density lipoprotein (HDL), and lower cardiovascular risk levels than adults not involved in the program.

_______________ 7. Time on the operating table, diastolic blood pressure, age, and preoperative albumin levels are related to development of pressure ulcers in hospitalized elderly.

_______________ 8. There are no differences in complications or incidence of phlebitis in heparin locks changed every 72 hours and those locks left in place up to 168 hours.

_______________ 9. Nurses' perceived work stress, internal locus of control, and social support are related to their psychological symptoms.

_______________ 10. Cancer patients with chronic pain who listen to music with positive suggestion of pain reduction have less pain than those who do not listen to music.

11. State hypothesis #5 as a null hypothesis.

12. State hypothesis #2 as a directional hypothesis.

13. State hypothesis # 9 as a null hypothesis.

EXERCISES IN CRITIQUE

Directions: Review the Carey et al. (2002) article in Appendix B and answer the following questions.

1. Are objectives, questions, or hypotheses stated in this study? ____________________
   Identify these.

2. Are these appropriate and clearly stated? Provide a rationale.

Directions: Review the Lewis et al. (1997) article in Appendix B and answer the following questions.

1. Are objectives, questions, or hypotheses stated in this study? ____________________
   Identify these.

2. Are these appropriate and clearly stated? Provide a rationale.

Directions: Review the Bruce and Grove (1994) article in Appendix B and answer the following questions.

1. Are objectives, questions, or hypotheses stated in this study? ____________________ Identify these.

2. Are these appropriate and clearly stated? Provide a rationale.

MAKING CONNECTIONS

Understanding Study Variables

Directions: Match each type of variable with the example variables provided below.

a. Demographic variable
b. Dependent variable
c. Independent variable

_____ 1. Age
_____ 2. Perception of pain
_____ 3. Exercise program
_____ 4. Gender
_____ 5. Length of hospital stay
_____ 6. Incidence of phlebitis
_____ 7. Relaxation therapy
_____ 8. Low-back massage
_____ 9. Educational level
_____ 10. Postoperative pain
_____ 11. Ethnic background
_____ 12. Marital status

EXERCISES IN CRITIQUE

Directions: Read the Carey et al. (2002) article and answer the following questions.

1. List the major variables in this study and identify the type of each variable (independent, dependent, or research).

Type of Variable	Variable

2. Identify the conceptual and operational definitions for the parenting stress and behavioral and emotional development.

3. Are these definitions clear? Provide a rationale.

Directions: Read the Lewis et al. (1997) article and answer the following questions.

1. List the variables in this article and identify the type of each variable (independent, dependent, or research).

Type of Variable	**Variable**

2. Identify the conceptual and operational definitions for the variable body position (right or left lateral).

3. Are these definitions clear? Provide a rationale.

Directions: Read the Bruce and Grove (1994) article and answer the following questions.

1. List the major variables in this article and identify the type of each variable (independent, dependent, or research).

Type of Variable	Variable

2. Identify the conceptual and operational definitions for the C.A.R.E. program variable.

3. Are these definitions clear? Provide a rationale.

chapter 4 Review of Literature

INTRODUCTION

You need to read Chapter 4 and then complete the following exercises. These exercises will assist you in reading and critiquing research reports and summarizing the findings for use in practice.

RELEVANT TERMS

Directions: Match each term below with its correct definition.

a. Academic library
b. Link
c. Computer search
d. Keywords
e. Full-text database
f. Dissertation
g. Empirical literature
h. Benchmarking
i. Integrative review of research
j. Interlibrary loan department
k. Primary source
l. Review of literature
m. Secondary source
n. Special library
o. Thesis
p. Complex search
q. Theoretical literature
r. Bibliographic database

Definitions

_____ 1. Source whose author summarizes or quotes content from a primary source.
_____ 2. Department that locates books and articles in other libraries and provides the sources within a designated time.
_____ 3. A search strategy that combines two or more keywords in one search.
_____ 4. Literature that includes concept analyses, conceptual maps, theories, and conceptual frameworks that support a selected research problem and purpose.
_____ 5. An electronic collection of complete journal articles.
_____ 6. Source whose author originated or is responsible for generating the ideas published.

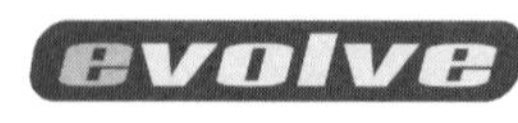

Be sure to check out the free exercises on-line at http://evolve.elsevier.com/Burns/understanding

_____ 7. Library that contains a collection of materials on a specific topic or specialty area, such as a library associated with a hospital.

_____ 8. Major concepts of a topic used to begin a computer search.

_____ 9. Review conducted to identify, analyze, and synthesize the results from independent studies to determine the current knowledge in a particular area.

_____ 10. Function conducted to scan the citations in different databases and identify sources relevant to a selected topic.

_____ 11. Review of theoretical and empirical sources to generate a picture of what is known and not known about a problem that provides a basis of the study conducted.

_____ 12. A research project completed by a student as part of the requirements for a master's degree.

_____ 13. A compilation of citations.

_____ 14. The results of meta-analyses that are used to establish a standard of quality care.

_____ 15. Relevant studies published in journals and books; also includes unpublished studies such as master's theses and doctoral dissertations.

_____ 16. Library located within an institution of higher learning that contains numerous journals and books.

_____ 17. Moves you from one Web site to another Web site.

_____ 18. An extensive, usually original research project that is completed by a doctoral student as part of the requirements for a doctoral degree.

KEY IDEAS

Directions: Fill in the blanks with the appropriate word(s).

1. Predominately two types of sources are reviewed and cited in a literature review; these are ______________________________ and __________________________ sources.
2. The purpose for conducting a literature review in phenomenological research is to ____.
3. The review of literature is conducted to provide a background for the conduct of a study in ______________________ and ________________________ studies.
4. The literature is reviewed to develop research questions and is a source of data in ____.

5. Williams' (1972) study, conducted to examine factors that contribute to skin breakdown, is considered a ______________________________ study in the area of pressure ulcer prevention.
6. A literature review should include what is ____________ and ______________ about the study problem.
7. Current sources for a literature review are defined as those that are ____________ ____.
8. This textbook, *Understanding Nursing Research,* is an example or a primary or secondary source? ____
9. Today, good libraries provide access to large numbers of ______________ ______________ that supply a broad scope of the available literature nationally and internationally.
10. Authorized users can access many library services at anytime and location through the ______________.
11. A written plan of a search strategy for a literature review should include:
    a.
    b.
    c.
    d.
12. The most relevant database for nursing literature is ______________.
13. Most electronic databases have a ________________ that can be used to identify keyword search terms.
14. Reference management software is used to ______________________________.
15. The yearly hardbound publication __________________________________ is a good source for integrative reviews of research relevant to nursing practice.
16. Reviewing the literature requires a ____________________________ of research sources to determine what is known and not known about a clinical problem.
17. The review of literature for use of study findings in practice usually includes the following sections: ____________________, ____________________ ________________________, and ______________________.

18. Sample research problem: "Although core rewarming is initiated prior to removal from the cardiopulmonary bypass machine (CPB), severe peripheral hypothermia and vasoconstriction often persist into the postoperative period" [Giuffre, M., Heidenreich, T., & Pruitt, L. (1994). Rewarming cardiac surgery patients: Radiant heat versus forced warm air. *Nursing Research, 43*(3), p. 174]. What keywords would you use to direct your review of literature for this problem?

19. Sample research problem: "Urinary incontinence is a common problem among nursing home (NH) residents and can be successfully treated with prompted voiding during daytime hours . . . Nighttime incontinence care should be individualized to minimize sleep disruption while considering moisture exposure that could affect skin health. Although descriptive studies have been published, there are no published intervention studies describing attempts to improve nighttime environmental factors in NHs" (p. 197) [Schnelle, J. F., Cruise, P. A., Alessi, C. A., Al-Samarrai, N., & Ouslander, J. G. (1998). Individualizing nighttime incontinence care in nursing home residents. *Nursing Research, 47*(4), 197-204]. What keywords would you use to direct your review of literature for this problem?

20. A search for existing literature related to a study problem requires multiple searches using various electronic databases. A written search record should be kept of searches performed that includes:

    a.

    b.

    c.

    d.

    e.

MAKING CONNECTIONS

Theoretical and Empirical Sources

Directions: Theoretical and empirical literature are included in the literature review of a published study. Read the sources below and label them with a **T** if they are theoretical sources or an **E** if they are empirical sources.

_____ 1. Lazarus and Folkman's Theory of Coping
_____ 2. Abstracts from a research conference
_____ 3. Theses
_____ 4. Watson's philosophy of human caring
_____ 5. Orem, D. E. (1991). *Nursing: Concepts of practice* (4th ed.) St. Louis: Mosby.
_____ 6. Giuffre, M., Heidenreich, T., & Pruitt, L. (1994). Rewarming cardiac surgery patients: Radiant heat versus forced warm air. *Nursing Research, 43*(3), 174–178.
_____ 7. Lowry, L. W., & Beikirch, P. (1998). Effects of comprehensive care on pregnancy outcomes. *Applied Nursing Research, 11*(2), 55-61.
_____ 8. Dissertations
_____ 9. von Bertalanffy, L. (1968). *General systems theory*. New York: Braziller.
_____ 10. Lewin's Change Theory
_____ 11. Burns, N., Carney, K., & Slinkman, C. (1998). Development of the rural-urban demand indicator. *Research in Nursing & Health, 21*(5), 453-466.

Primary and Secondary Sources

Directions: A literature review includes mainly primary sources. Label the sources below with a **P** if they are primary sources or an **S** if they are secondary sources.

_____ 1. Integrated review of research
_____ 2. Dissertations
_____ 3. Theses
_____ 4. Textbooks
_____ 5. Summary of theoretical and empirical sources
_____ 6. Study published in *Applied Nursing Research*
_____ 7. Landmark study of pressure ulcers
_____ 8. Published review of literature article
_____ 9. Exact replication of a study
_____ 10. Historical research article in *Image: Journal of Nursing Scholarship*

EXERCISES IN CRITIQUE

Directions: Review the three articles in Appendix B and use these articles to answer the following questions.

1. The most common way to cite a reference is the American Psychological Association (APA) (2001) format. Knowing the different parts of a reference citation will assist you in locating and recording sources for a formal paper. The following source is presented in APA format.

   Bruce, S. L., & Grove, S. K. (1994). The effect of a coronary artery risk evaluation program on serum lipid values and cardiovascular risk levels. *Applied Nursing Research, 7*(2), 67–74.

   a. In this reference, *Applied Nursing Research* is the ________________.
   b. In this reference, the 1994 is ________________________________.
   c. In this reference, the 7 is ______________________________.
   d. In this reference, the 67–74 is ___________________________.
   e. In this reference, the 2 is ______________________________.
   f. Who are the authors of this article? ________________ and ________________
   g. What is the title of the article? ____

   ____

2. Write the reference for the Carey, Nicholson, and Fox (2002) article using APA format.

 ____

 ____

 ____

3. If the reference citations below are not complete, indicate what is missing. Incomplete references in published studies are a problem for individuals trying to locate sources from the reference list of the article.
   a. Christman, S. K., Fish, A. F., Frid, D. J., Smith, B. A., & Bryant, C. X. (1998). *Applied Nursing Research, 7*(2).
   What is missing?

   b. Anderson, M. A., & Helms, L. B. (1998). Extended care referral after hospital discharge. *Research in Nursing & Health,* (5).
   What is missing?

   c. Schlenk, E. A., & Boehm, S. Behaviors in type II diabetes during contingency contracting. *Applied Nursing Research,* 77-83.
   What is missing?

4. What are the titles for the literature review section in the three articles in Appendix B?
   a. Carey, Nicholson, & Fox (2002) ______________________
   b. Lewis, Nichols, Mackey, Fadol, Sloane, Villagomez, & Liehr (1997) __________
   ____
   c. Bruce & Grove (1994) ______________________

5. Are relevant studies identified and described in the Carey et al. (2002) literature review? Give examples of two studies that are cited in the literature review of the article.

6. Are relevant theories identified and described in the Carey et al. (2002) study? Identify one theoretical source that is cited in the study's literature review.

7. In Carey et al. (2002) study references, is the source by Fox, Platz, and Bentley (1995) a primary or secondary source? ______________________________

8. Is there a source in the References section of the Carey et al. (2002) study that is an integrated review of the literature?

9. Are the references in Carey et al. (2002) study current? Provide a rationale.

10. Does the literature review in Carey et al. (2002) study present the current knowledge base for the research problem? Provide a rationale.

11. Are relevant studies identified and described in the Lewis et al. (1997) study? Give examples of two studies that are cited in the literature review of the article.

12. Are relevant theories identified and described in the Lewis et al. (1997) study? Identify one theoretical source that is cited in the study's literature review.

13. In Lewis et al. (1997) study references, is the source by Luckmann and Sorensen (1993) a primary or secondary source? ____________________________ Is the source by Shinners and Pease (1993) a primary or secondary source? ___________________

14. Are the references in Lewis et al. (1997) study current? Provide a rationale.

15. Does the literature review in Lewis et al. (1997) study provide a current knowledge base for the research problem examined in this study?

16. Are relevant studies identified and described in the Bruce and Grove (1994) study? Give examples of two studies that are cited in the literature review of the article.

17. Are relevant theories identified and described in the Bruce and Grove (1994) study? Identify one theoretical source that is cited in the study's literature review.

18. In Bruce and Grove's references, is the source by Glanz (1988) a primary or secondary source? ______________________________ Is the source by Blair, Bryant, and Bocuzzi (1988) a primary or secondary source? ______________________________

19. Are the references in Bruce and Grove's (1994) study current? Provide a rationale.

20. Does the literature review of Bruce and Grove's (1994) study provide the current knowledge base of the problem examined in this study? Provide a rationale.

GOING BEYOND

1. Identify a problem in clinical practice and conduct a summary of the research literature on this topic.

    a. Search the literature for relevant research sources. Has an integrative review been done on this topic?

    b. Locate relevant studies in your university library.

    c. Read each study and identify the steps of the research process.

    d. Outline key information from each study including the study purpose, frame work, sample size, design, results, and findings.

    e. Critique the quality of each study.

    f. Write a description of each research report and critique the quality of the report.

    g. Then write a summary paragraph that indicates what is known and not known about your clinical problem.

    h. Ask your instructor to evaluate your review of the research literature.

chapter 5 Understanding Theory and Research Frameworks

INTRODUCTION

You need to read Chapter 5 and then complete the following exercises. These exercises will assist you in learning relevant terms and identifying and critiquing frameworks in published studies.

RELEVANT TERMS

Directions: Define the following terms in your own words without looking at your textbook. Then check your definitions with those in the glossary of your textbook. Using this strategy, you can identify elements of the term that are not yet clear in your mind. Reread that section of the chapter to clarify your understanding of the term.

Abstract ____

____

Concept ____

____

Conceptual definition ____

____

Concrete ____

____

Conceptual model ____

____

Construct ____

____

Existence statement ____

____

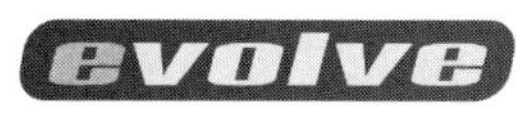

Be sure to check out the free exercises on-line at http://evolve.elsevier.com/Burns/understanding

Hypotheses ____

____

Relational statement ____

____

Proposition____

____

Theory ____

____

Variable____

____

KEY IDEAS

Directions: Fill in the blanks in this section with the appropriate word(s) or numbers.

1. We use theories to ______________________________.
2. Testing a theory involves ______________________________.
3. ______________________ are not generally considered testable.
4. Research is based on ______________________.
5. A framework that has been used rather shallowly to provide an overall orientation for a study but does not guide the study is referred to as __________________.
6. Research findings are interpreted in terms of ______________________.
7. In a framework, all ______________________ should be defined.
8. Concepts in conceptual models are referred to as ______________________.
9. A ______________ is more specific than a concept and is defined so that it is measurable.
10. The ______________________ of a theory are tested through research.
11. Statements at the lowest level of abstraction are referred to as ______________.
12. The purpose of a conceptual map is to ______________________________ ____.
13. A conceptual map includes ______________________________ ____.

14. An organized program of research designed to build a body of knowledge related to a particular conceptual model is referred to as a ______________________.

MAKING CONNECTIONS

Directions: Match the following ideas.

____	1. Theory	a.	Broadly explains phenomena of interest
____	2. Concept	b.	The basic element of a theory
____	3. Conceptual model	c.	Expresses a claim important to a theory
____	4. Variable	d.	Graphically shows interrelations among concepts
____	5. Statement		
____	6. Conceptual map	e.	Integrated set of defined concepts and statements
____	7. Framework		
____	8. Construct	f.	Statement expressed at low level of abstraction
____	9. Hypothesis	g.	Provides general meanings of terms
		h.	Defines a term so that it is measurable
		i.	Presents portions of a theory to be tested in a study

EXERCISES IN CRITIQUE

Directions: Examine the framework of Lewis, Nichols, Mackey, Fadol, Sloane, Villagomez, and Liehr's study in Appendix B and answer the following questions.

1. List the concepts in the study.

2. State the definition of each concept as defined by the author(s). Are the definitions clear and adequate? If not, identify the inadequacies.

3. Complete the following table for the Lewis et al. (1997) study by listing each concept, its related variable(s), and measurement method.

Concept	Variable	Measurement

4. Compare the measurement method for each variable with its associated concept and conceptual definition. Is each measurement method consistent with its associated concept and conceptual definition? If not, identify any inconsistencies?

5. List the statements expressed within the publication. Underline the concepts included in each statement. Are all of the study concepts included within a statement? Provide a map of each statement.

6. State the proposition(s) being tested in the Lewis et al. (1997) study and their related hypothesis or research question.

7. Are the statements tested by the study design? How?

8. Is the framework expressed as a conceptual map? Are all of the concepts in the study included in the map? Are all of the statements you identified included in the map? If there is no map, develop one and draw it here.

9. Does the author provide statements for each linkage between concepts shown on the map? Does the author provide references from the literature to support the linkages? List the references for each linkage.

10. Develop a short summary paragraph describing the strengths and weaknesses of the framework.

GOING BEYOND

The framework of Carey, Nicholson, and Fox (2002) is expressed as a Conceptual Model. Unlike the model of Lewis, et al., their framework includes concepts and is more abstract. They do not provide a conceptual map. Using their theoretical statements, go through the Exercises in Critique on the previous pages, addressing each item in terms of the Carey, et al. study.

The framework for Bruce & Grove's study was removed by the editors prior to publication. Try to construct a framework for their study from the introduction and literature review.

chapter 6 Examining Ethics in Nursing Research

INTRODUCTION

You need to read Chapter 6 and then complete the following exercises. These exercises will assist you in understanding the ethical aspects of studies. The answers for these exercises are in Appendix A under Chapter 6.

RELEVANT TERMS

Directions: Match each term below with its correct definition.

a. Anonymity
b. Benefit-risk ratio
c. Confidentiality
d. Discomfort and harm
e. Ethical principles
f. Human rights
g. Informed consent
h. Institutional review
i. Nontherapeutic research
j. Privacy Act
k. Scientific misconduct
l. Therapeutic research

Definitions

_____ 1. Claims and demands that have been justified in the eyes of an individual or by the consensus of a group of individuals and are protected in research.

_____ 2. Condition in which a subject's identity cannot be linked, even by the researcher, with his or her individual responses.

_____ 3. Agreement by a prospective subject to voluntarily participate in a study after he or she has assimilated essential information about the study.

_____ 4. Research conducted to generate knowledge for a discipline; the results might benefit future patients but will probably not benefit the research subjects.

_____ 5. Process of examining studies for ethical concerns by a committee of peers.

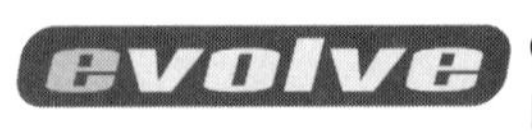

Be sure to check out the free exercises on-line at http://evolve.elsevier.com/Burns/understanding

_____ 6. Phrase used to describe the degree of risk for a subject participating in a study. This level of risk includes no anticipated effects, temporary discomfort, unusual levels of temporary discomfort, risk of permanent damage, or certainty of permanent damage.

_____ 7. Freedom of an individual to determine the time, extent, and general circumstances under which private information will be shared with or withheld from others.

_____ 8. Ratio considered by researchers and reviewers of research as they weigh potential benefits and risks in a study to promote the conduct of ethical research.

_____ 9. Research that provides a patient with an opportunity to receive an experimental treatment that might have beneficial results.

_____ 10. Principles of respect for persons, beneficence, and justice that are relevant to the conduct of research.

_____ 11. Management of private data in research in such a way that subjects' identities are not linked with their responses.

_____ 12. Practices such as fabrication, falsification, or forging of data; dishonest manipulation of the study design or methods; and plagiarism.

KEY IDEAS

Directions: Fill in the blanks with the correct responses.

1. The elements of informed consent include:

   a. ______________________________

   b. ______________________________

   c. ______________________________

   d. ______________________________

2. Identify six types of information that must be included in the consent form.

   a. ______________________________

   b. ______________________________

   c. ______________________________

   d. ______________________________

   e. ______________________________

   f. ______________________________

3. ______________________ consent means that the prospective subject has decided to take part in a study of his or her own volition without coercion or any undue influence.
4. Subjects with diminished autonomy (e.g., the mentally ill or children) are vulnerable and ______________________ to consent to participate in research.
5. Before a study is conducted, it must be reviewed by a committee of peers, which is called an ______________________.
6. The three levels of institutional review of research are:
   a. ______________________
   b. ______________________
   c. ______________________
7. How do you assess the benefit-risk ratio of a published study?

8. What type of institutional review would a study probably require if it involved the review of patients' records to identify their fasting blood glucose value prior to surgery? ______________________
9. A study that involved examining the effects of a new drug on patients' serum lipid values would probably require what type of institutional review? ______________________
10. Identify three different types of scientific misconduct.
    a. ______________________
    b. ______________________
    c. ______________________
11. The names of the two federal agencies that were organized for reporting and investigating scientific misconduct are ______________________ and ______________________.

12. Is scientific misconduct present in nursing? ______________________________

13. Are animals used in research conducted by nurses? ________________________

14. What agency was developed to ensure the humane treatment of animals in research? ____

15. Should animals be used as research subjects? Provide a rationale for your response.

MAKING CONNECTIONS

Historical Events, Ethical Codes, and Regulations

Directions: Match the unethical studies listed below with the correct description.

a. Jewish Chronic Disease Hospital Study
b. Nazi Medical Experiments
c. Tuskegee Syphilis Study
d. Willowbrook Study

_____ 1. Subjects were exposed to freezing temperatures, high altitudes, poisons, untested drugs, and experimental operations.
_____ 2. Study was conducted to determine the natural course of syphilis in the adult black male.
_____ 3. Subjects were deliberately infected with the hepatitis virus in this study.
_____ 4. Subjects were frequently killed or sustained permanent physical, mental, or social damage during these studies.
_____ 5. Subjects did not receive penicillin when it was identified as an effective treatment for their disease.
_____ 6. The purpose of this study was to determine the patients' rejection responses to live cancer cells.
_____ 7. The subjects in this study were institutionalized, mentally retarded children.
_____ 8. These experiments resulted in the development of the Nuremberg Code.
_____ 9. The subjects were injected with live cancer cells without their knowledge.
____ 10. This study continued until 1972 when an account of the study appeared in the Washington Star and public outrage demanded the study be stopped.

PUZZLE

Directions: Complete the crossword puzzle below. Note that if the answer is more than one word, there are no blank spaces left between the words.

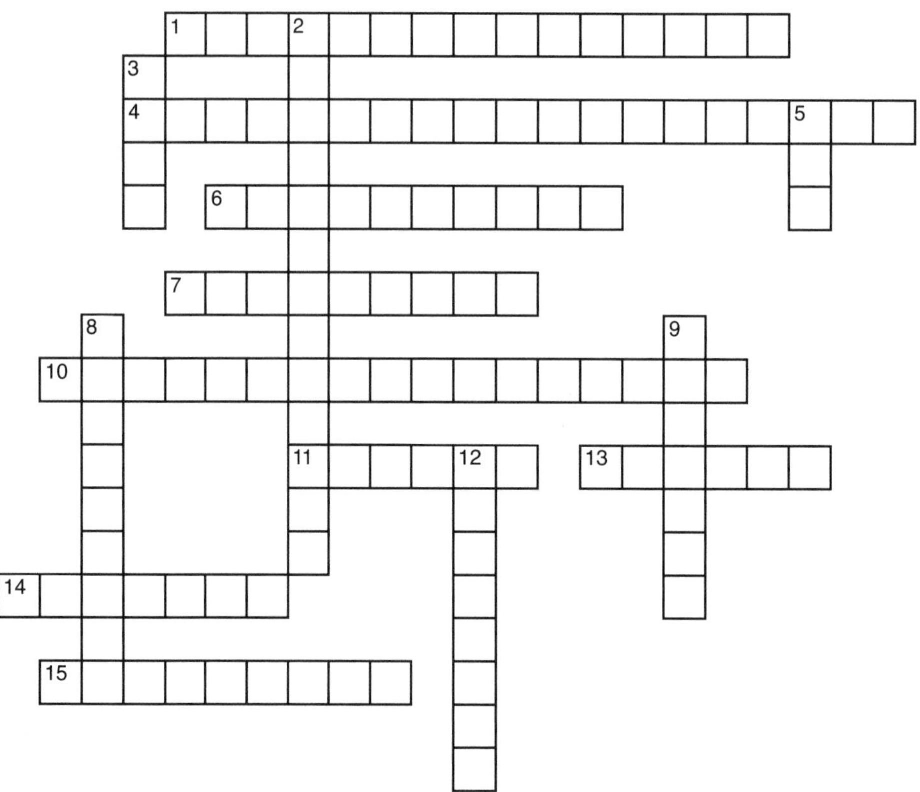

ACROSS

1. Keeping data private.
4. Agency evaluation of a study to protect potential subjects.
6. Subjects who can legally choose to participate or not in a study are _____.
7. Code developed after World War II.
10. Controlling your own fate.
11. Focuses on human rights of research.
13. Child's agreement to be in a study.
14. ____ act of 1974.
15. Identity of subjects unknown.

DOWN

2. Subject should receive ____ ____ during a study.
3. Opposite of benefit that must be examined to determine if a study is ethical.
5. Institutional Review Board.
8. Misinforming subjects.
9. Subject's permission to be in a study.
12. _____ are incompetent to give consent.

EXERCISES IN CRITIQUE

Directions: Review the research articles in Appendix B to answer the following questions.

1. Is the Carey, Nicholson, and Fox (2002) study ethical? Identify the information in the study that indicates the subjects' rights were protected and institutional review was obtained.

2. Is the Lewis, Nichols, Mackey, Fadol, Sloane, Villagomez, and Liehr (1997) study ethical? Identify the information in the study that indicates the subjects' rights were protected and institutional review was obtained.

3. Is the Bruce and Grove (1994) study ethical? Identify the information in the study that indicates the subjects' rights were protected and institutional review was obtained.

chapter 7 Clarifying Research Designs

INTRODUCTION

You need to read Chapter 7 and then complete the following exercises. These exercises will assist you in learning relevant terms and identifying and critiquing designs in published studies.

RELEVANT TERMS

Directions: Define the following terms in your own words without looking in your textbook. Then check your definitions with those in the glossary of your textbook. Using this strategy, you can identify elements of the term that are not yet clear in your mind. Reread that section of the chapter to clarify your understanding of the term.

Bias ____

____

Causality ____

____

Control ____

____

Design validity ____

____

External validity ____

____

Heterogeneity ____

____

Homogeneity ____

____

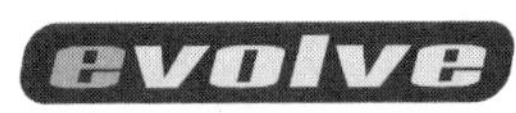

Be sure to check out the free exercises on-line at http://evolve.elsevier.com/Burns/understanding

Internal validity ____

____

Manipulation ____

____

Multicausality ____

____

Probability ____

____

KEY IDEAS

Directions: Fill in the blanks in this section with the appropriate word(s) or numbers.

1. According to causality theory, things have causes and causes lead to ______________.
2. From the perspective of probability, a _________ may not produce a specific __________ each time that particular ________________ occurs.
3. Designs are developed to reduce the possibilities and effects of ________________.
4. The purpose of research designs is to maximize ___________ factors in the study situation.
5. The most commonly used manipulation in a study is the ____________________.
6. Critical analysis of research involves being able to think through ________________ ____________ that have occurred and make judgments about how seriously these affect the integrity of the findings.
7. Quasi-experimental and experimental studies are designed to examine ______________________________________.
8. In most studies, ______________________ are the basis of obtaining valid answers.
9. Designs were developed to reduce threats to the validity of the _______________.

MAKING CONNECTIONS

Directions: Match each term below with its correct definition.

_____ 1. Design validity
_____ 2. Multicausality
_____ 3. Descriptive design
_____ 4. Bias
_____ 5. Control
_____ 6. Internal validity
_____ 7. Probability
_____ 8. External validity
_____ 9. Correlational design

a. To deviate from the true or expected.
b. The extent to which study findings can be generalized beyond the sample used in the study.
c. Extent to which the effects detected in the study are a true reflection of reality.
d. Addresses relative causality.
e. To examine relationships between or among two or more variables in a single group.
f. The power to direct or manipulate factors to achieve a desired outcome.
g. The study provides a convincing test of the framework propositions.
h. The recognition that a number of interrelating variables can be involved in causing a particular effect.
i. To gain more information about characteristics in a particular field of study.

Directions: Match each design type with the corresponding study description.

a. Typical descriptive study design
b. Comparative descriptive design
c. Longitudinal design
d. Trend design
e. Case study design
f. Descriptive correlational design
g. Predictive correlational design
h. Model testing design
i. Quasi-experimental design
j. Experimental design

_____ 1. The purpose of this study was to describe the physical status, emotional state (depression and motivation), and functional performance of residents in a long-term care facility and to explore the impact of motivation (intrinsic and extrinsic factors), demographic variables, length of time institutionalized, physical status, depression, and fear of falling on functional performance of older adults in a long-term care setting (Resnick, 1998, p. 231).

_____ 2. Annual self-assessments of MS [multiple sclerosis]-related symptoms and level of ADL [activities of daily living] functioning were used to examine the chronic ilness trajectory over a 10-year period (Gulick, 1998, p. 138).

_____ 3. The purpose of the study was to describe the relationships among perceived social support, uncertainty, and psychological distress in adolescents recently diagnosed with cancer (Neville, 1998, p. 38).

_____ 4. The purpose of this study is to examine patient characteristics that predict referral to outpatient CR [cardiac rehabilitation] following hospitalization for MI [myocardial infarction] or CABG [coronary artery bypass surgery] (Burns, Camaione, Froman, & Clark, 1998, p. 148).

_____ 5. The purpose of this study was to describe and compare differences in demographics, prenatal care use, and pregnancy, labor, postpartum, and neonatal complications for 129 pregnant Mexican-American adolescents who were either born in the United States or born in Mexico (Koshar, Lee, Goss, Heilemann, & Stinson, 1998).

_____ 6. The purpose of the study was to examine the effects of ovarian hormone cessation, hormone supplementation, and dietary fiber composition on body weight, appetite, and intestinal transit. In Part 1, effects of ovarian hormone status on body weight and baseline and stimulated intestinal transit were measured in chow-fed rats. Sprague-Dawley rats were ovariectomized (OVX), then injected daily (22 days) with estrogen (E), progesterone (P), the combination (E+P), or placebo. Controls were sham operated and placebo injected (Bond, Heitkemper, & Jarrett, 1994, p. 18).

_____ 7. The purpose of this study was to describe and analyze events occurring to a single patient who experienced hypokalemic periodic paralysis (Anderson, 1998).

_____ 8. The purpose of this study was to compare the safety of automatic blood pressure cuffs versus manual cuffs when used on patients receiving thrombolytic therapy. This prospective, randomized trial compared manual and automatic devices for measuring blood pressure. A convenience sample was used to study patients in eight hospitals throughout the United States (Saul, Smith, & Mook, 1998, p. 193).

_____ 9. The purpose of this study was to develop and examine the predictive ability of a model of exercise among older adults (Conn, 1998, p. 180).

_____ 10. This paper shows the infant mortality rates (IMR) for all of Queensland, and at Cherbourg from 1910 to 1990 and the weights of four cohorts of children at Cherbourg over 40 years (Alsop-Shields 1998).

Mapping the Design

Directions: Map the design for the following quasi-experimental studies.

1. The purpose of the study was to investigate the effects of a transmural home care intervention program for terminal cancer patients on the direct caregivers' (the patient's principal informal caregiver) quality of life, compared with standard care programs. The intervention program intended to optimize the cooperation and coordination between the intramural and extramural health care organizations (transmural care). Direct caregivers of terminal cancer patients (estimated prognosis of less than 6 months) could be included in this quasi-experimental study. The direct caregivers' quality of life was measured in a multidimensional way 1 week before (T1), 1 week after (T2), and 4 weeks after (T3) the patient's discharge from the hospital (discharge being the starting point of the intervention), then again at 3 months after the patient's death (T4) (Smeenk, de Witte, van Haastragt, Schipper, Beizemans, & Crebolder, 1998, p. 129) . . . Direct caregivers of patients fulfilling the inclusion criteria and living in Eindhoven, The Netherlands, were allocated to the intervention group and those living in the urban surroundings of Eindhoven were allocated to the control group. After the patients' discharge from the hospital (i.e., the start of the intervention), patients and their direct caregivers in both groups received the standard care available in The Netherlands (Schrijvers, 1997). In addition to this care, patients and their direct caregivers allocated to the intervention group were offered the intervention program (p. 130).

2. Objectives: To test a structured communications program for family members to determine whether the program would increase family members' satisfaction with care, meet their needs for information better, and decrease disruption for the ICU nursing staff caused by incoming telephone calls from patients' family members (p. 24) . . . The groups consisted of family members of patients in a medical ICU. Only one medical ICU was used, so that the setting and personnel would not differ between the two groups. The experimental group received the structured communication program, and the control group received usual care. Pretest data were collected approximately 24 hours after the patient was admitted to the medical ICU. Posttest data were collected on the day of discharge from the unit or 2 weeks after admission to the unit for those patients who had not been discharged yet. The same instruments were administered before and after the intervention (pretest and posttest) to both groups. To prevent contamination between groups, we collected data for the control group first. After the control-group phase was finished, the nature of the intervention was explained to the ICU nurses and the intervention phase was started (Medland, Ferrans, & the College of Nursing, University of Illinois at Chicago, 1998, p. 25).

EXERCISES IN CRITIQUE

Directions: Review the research articles in Appendix B and answer the following questions.

1. Identify the design used in:
   a. Carey and colleagues' study ______________________
   b. Lewis and colleagues' study ______________________
   c. Bruce and Grove's study ______________________

2. Identify three sources of potential bias in the study design of:

   a. Carey and colleagues' study ______________________
   ____
   ____

   b. Lewis and colleagues' study ______________________
   ____
   ____

   c. Bruce and Grove's study ______________________
   ____
   ____

3. List three methods of control used in the design of:

   a. Carey and colleagues' study ______________________
   ____
   ____

   b. Lewis and colleagues' study ______________________
   ____
   ____

c. Bruce and Grove's study ____

____

____

4. What comparisons could be made, given the design used in:

a. Carey and colleagues' study

b. Lewis and colleagues' study

c. Bruce and Grove's study

5. To what populations can the findings be generalized from:

a. Carey and colleagues' study

b. Lewis and colleagues' study

c. Bruce and Grove's study

6. What are the threats to external validity in:

   a. Carey and colleagues' study

   b. Lewis and colleagues' study

   c. Bruce and Grove's study

7. Identify three strengths in the design used by:

   a. Carey and colleagues ______________________________

   ____

   ____

   b. Lewis and colleagues ______________________________

   ____

   ____

   c. Bruce and Grove ______________________________

   ____

   ____

GOING BEYOND

Examine the relationships among the study framework; research objectives, questions, or hypotheses; and design in the three studies in Appendix B.

1. Does the design allow an adequate test of the research objectives, questions, or hypotheses?

2. Does the design facilitate application of the findings to the framework?

References

Alsop-Shields, L. (1998). Changes in transcultural nursing and its influence on the growth of Australian Aboriginal children. *Journal of Pediatric Nursing, 13*(2), 119–126.

Anderson, K. M. (1998). Hypokalemic periodic paralysis: A case study. *American Journal of Critical Care, 7*(3), 236–239.

Bond, E. F., Heitkemper, M. M., & Jarrett, M. (1994). Intestinal transit and body weight responses to ovarian hormones and dietary fiber in rats. *Nursing Research, 43*(1), 18–24.

Burns, K. J., Camaione, D. N., Froman, R. D., & Clark, B. A. III. (1998). Predictors of referral to cardiac rehabilitation and cardiac exercise self-efficacy. *Clinical Nursing Research, 7*(2), 147–163.

Burns, S. M., Marshall, M., Burns, J. E., Ryan, B., Wilmoth, D., Carpenter, R., Aloi, A., Wood, M., & Truwit, J. D. (1998). Design, testing, and results of an outcomes-managed approach to patients requiring prolonged mechanical ventilation. *American Journal of Critical Care, 7*(1), 45–57).

Koshar, J. H., Lee, K. A., Goss, G., Heilemann, M. S., & Stinson, J. (1998). The Hispanic teen mother's origin of birth, use of prenatal care, and maternal and neonatal complications. *Journal of Pediatric Nursing, 13*(3), 151–157.

Medland, J. J., Ferrans, C. E., & the College of Nursing, University of Illinois at Chicago (1998). Effectiveness of a structured communication program for family members of patients in an ICU. *American Journal of Critical Care, 7*(1), 24–29.

Neville, K. (1998). The relationships among uncertainty, social support, and psychological distress in adolescents recently diagnosed with cancer. *Journal of Pediatric Oncology Nursing, 15*(1), 37–46.

Schrijvers, A. J. P. (1997). *Health and health care in The Netherlands. A critical self-assessment by Dutch experts in the medical and health sciences.* Utrecht: De Tijdstroom B. V.

Smeenk, F. W. J. M., de Witte, L. P., van Haastregt, J. C. M., Schipper, R. M., Biezemans, H. P. H., & Creboler, H. F. J. M. (1998). Transmural care of terminal cancer patients: Effects on the quality of life of direct caregivers. *Nursing Research, 47*(3), 129–136.

chapter 8 Populations and Samples

INTRODUCTION

You need to read Chapter 8 and then complete the following exercises. These exercises will assist you in understanding the sampling process in published studies. The answers to these exercises are in Appendix A under Chapter 8.

RELEVANT TERMS

Directions: Match each term below with its correct definition.

a. Accessible population
b. Cluster sampling
c. Convenience sampling
d. Network sampling
e. Nonprobability sampling
f. Probability sampling
g. Purposive sampling
h. Quote sampling
i. Random sampling
j. Sampling
k. Sampling criteria
l. Stratified random sampling
m. Systematic sampling
n. Target population

Definitions

_____ 1. Process of selecting a group of people, events, behaviors, or other elements that are representative of the population being studied.
_____ 2. Portion of the target population to which the researcher has reasonable access.
_____ 3. All elements (individuals, objects, events, or substances) that meet the sample criteria for inclusion in a study.
_____ 4. Judgmental sampling that involves the conscious selection by the researcher of certain subjects or elements to include in a study.
_____ 5. List of the characteristics essential for membership in the target population.

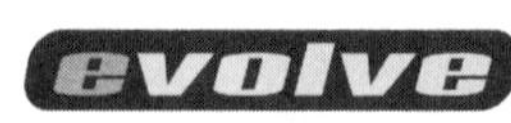

Be sure to check out the free exercises on-line at http://evolve.elsevier.com/Burns/understanding

_____ 6. Random sampling technique in which every member (element) of the population has a probability higher than zero of being selected for the sample; examples include simple random sampling, stratified random sampling, cluster sampling, and systematic sampling.

_____ 7. Sampling technique selecting every kth individual from an ordered list of all members of a population, using a random selected starting point.

_____ 8. Random selection of subjects from the sampling frame for a study.

_____ 9. Random sampling technique used when the researcher knows some of the variables in the population that are critical to achieving representativeness; the sample is divided into strata or groups using these identified variables.

_____ 10. Sampling technique in which a frame is developed that includes a list of all states, cities, institutions, or organizations (clusters) that could be used in a study; a randomized sample is drawn from this list.

_____ 11. Snowballing technique that takes advantage of social networks and the fact that friends tend to hold characteristics in common; subjects meeting sample criteria are asked to assist in locating others with similar characteristics.

_____ 12. Sampling in which not every element of the population has an opportunity for selection, such as convenience sampling, quota sampling, purposive sampling, and network sampling.

_____ 13. Convenience sampling technique with an added strategy to ensure the inclusion of subjects who are likely to be underrepresented in the convenience sample, such as women and minority groups.

_____ 14. Sampling technique that involves including subjects in a study because they happened to be in the right place at the right time.

KEY IDEAS

Directions: Fill in the blanks with the appropriate word(s).

1. The individual units of a population are called ______________________________.
2. The sample is obtained from the accessible population and is generalized to the ____.
3. Representativeness means that the ____________________, ____________________ ______________________, and ____ are alike in as many ways as possible.

4. Identify two ways you might evaluate the representativeness of a sample in a published study.

   a. ______________________________

   b. ______________________________

5. Random variation is ______________________________.

6. A list of every member of a population is referred to as a ______________________________.

7. Sampling plan outlines the ______________________________.

8. In critiquing the sampling plan in a study, what three things might you examine?

   a. ______________________________

   b. ______________________________

   c. ______________________________

9. When the sampling criteria are narrowly defined or very specific, the sample desired is ______________________________.

10. When the sampling criteria are broadly defined to include a variety of subjects, the sample desired is______________________________.

11. Subjects must be over the age of 18, able to read and write English, newly diagnosed with cancer, and have no other major illnesses. These are examples of ______________________________.

12. The sample was 65% female and 40% African American, 30% Hispanic, and 30% Caucasian, which are examples of ______________________________.

13. When subjects are lost to the study, this is referred to as ______________________________.

14. The term *control group* is limited to only those studies using ______________________________ sampling methods.

15. If ______________________________ sampling methods are used for sample selection, the group not receiving the treatment is referred to as a comparison group.

16. Identify four types of probability sampling.
    a. ______________________________
    b. ______________________________
    c. ______________________________
    d. ______________________________

17. When subjects are randomly selected and then randomly assigned to treatment or control groups, this is a ____________________ sampling technique.
18. Identify four types of nonprobability sampling.
    a. ______________________________
    b. ______________________________
    c. ______________________________
    d. ______________________________
19. Currently, do the majority of nursing studies use probability or nonprobability sampling methods? ____________________
20. Convenience sampling is also called ____________________.
21. Purposive sampling is referred to as ____________________.
22. The adequacy of the sample size can be evaluated using ____________________ ____________________.
23. Power is the capacity to detect ____________________ or ____________________ that actually exist in the population.
24. The minimal acceptable level of power for a study is ____________.
25. If the findings of a study are nonsignificant, the researcher should examine the adequacy of the sample size by running a ____________________.
26. Effect size is the extent to which the ____________________ is false.
27. Identify five factors that influence the adequacy of a study's sample size.
    a. ______________________________
    b. ______________________________
    c. ______________________________
    d. ______________________________
    e. ______________________________

MAKING CONNECTIONS

Directions: Match the sampling method with the examples of sampling methods from published studies. Some of the sampling methods might be used more than once.

a. Cluster sampling
b. Convenience sampling
c. Network sampling
d. Purposive sampling
e. Quota sampling
f. Simple random sampling
g. Stratified random sampling
h. Systematic sampling

_____ 1. A sample of 500 nurses were randomly selected from a list of all registered nurses in the state of Texas.

_____ 2. A-sample of 50 diabetic patients was obtained from an outpatient clinic and randomly placed in the comparison and experimental groups.

_____ 3. A sample of 10 HIV subjects was obtained by asking three subjects to identify their friends with HIV who might participate in the study.

_____ 4. A sample of 1000 critical care nurses was obtained by asking 100 critical care nurse managers in 50 randomly selected, large hospitals to identify 10 staff nurses to complete a survey.

_____ 5. A sample of 50 subjects were asked to participate in a study at an immunization booth in the mall.

_____ 6. Gender was used to stratify a sample of 100 randomly selected subjects.

_____ 7. The researcher obtained a list of all certified nurse practitioners, picked a random starting point, and then selected every 25th individual to participate in the study.

_____ 8. A sample of 50 hypertensive subjects were recruited in a clinic to participate in a study.

_____ 9. An equal number of patients with asthma, emphysema, and chronic bronchitis were recruited from the local Better Breathers Chapter to participate in a study.

_____ 10. The sample included 50 patients; 25 were examples of strong self-care and 25 were examples of poor self-care.

_____ 11. A sample of 5000 military personnel were randomly selected to participate in a study.

_____ 12. A sample of 10 drug-addicted nurses were obtained by asking five subjects to identify their friends who were drug-addicted.

_____ 13. A sample of 25 home health patients were asked to participate in a study because they had a history of pressure ulcers that would not heal.

_____ 14. A sample of 50 adolescents were obtained at a fast food place.

_____ 15. A sample of 50 surgery patients were randomly selected from a hospital and randomly placed in control and treatment groups.

PUZZLES

Directions: Complete the crossword puzzle on the next page. Note that if the answer is more than one word, there are no blank spaces left between the words.

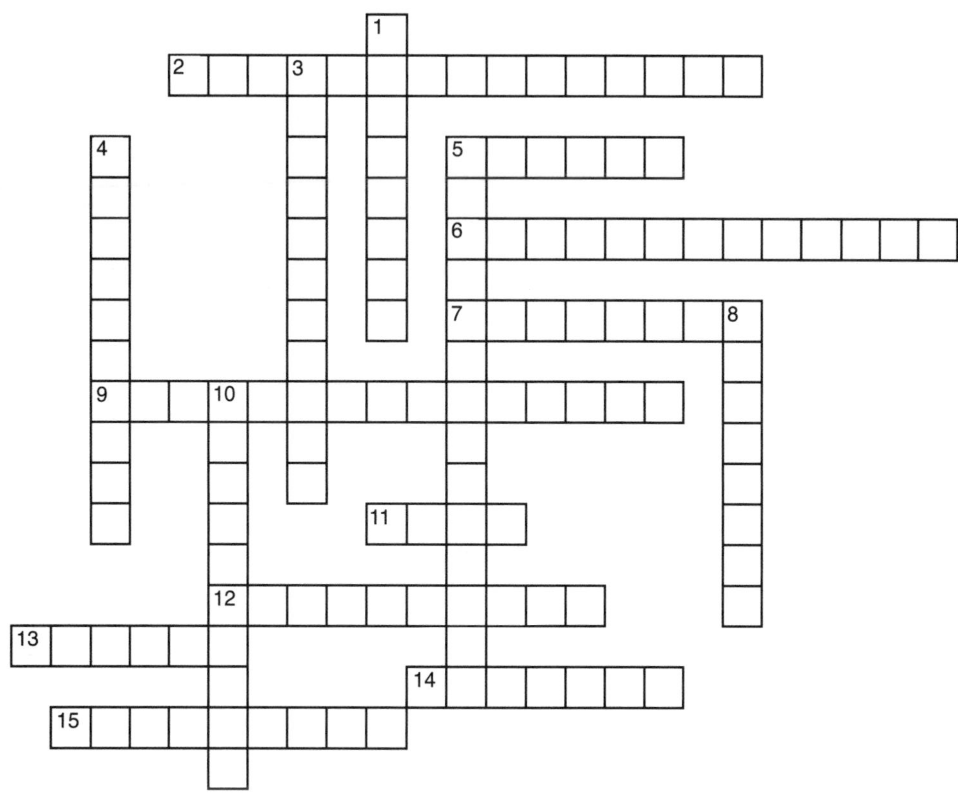

ACROSS

2. Group in a study.
5. Equal opportunity to be a subject.
6. Used to determine sample size.
7. Make up the population.
9. Used to select subjects.
11. Slanted from truth.
12. Population from which subjects are selected.
13. Population designated by sample criteria.
14. Possible sampling method used when studying subjects with HIV.
15. Nonprobability sampling method.

DOWN

1. Determines who is in a sample.
3. Random sampling.
4. Number of subjects in a study.
5. Sample is ____ of population.
8. People in a study.
10. Target ____.

EXERCISES IN CRITIQUE

Directions: Review the Bruce & Grove (1994) article in Appendix B and answer the following questions.

1. List the sample criteria for this study.

2. Identify the sample characteristics for this study.

3. What is the sample size? ______________ Was a power analysis used to determine the sample size? _________

4. Was the sample size adequate? Provide a rationale.

5. What was the sample mortality for this study?

6. Was probability or nonprobability sampling used in this study?

____

7. What specific type of sampling method was used in this study?

____

8. Was the sample in this study representative of the population studied? Provide a rationale.

9. Can the findings be generalized? Provide a rationale.

Directions: Review the Carey et al. study in Appendix B to answer the following questions.

1. List the sample criteria for this study.

2. Identify the sample characteristics for this study.

3. What is the sample size? ______________

4. Was the sample size adequate? Provide a rationale.

5. What was the sample mortality for this study?

6. Was probability or nonprobability sampling used in this study?

   ____

7. What specific type of sampling method was used in this study?

   ____

8. Was the sample in this study representative of the population studied? Provide a rationale.

9. Can the findings be generalized? Provide a rationale.

Directions: Review the Lewis et al. study in Appendix B to answer the following questions.

1. List the sample criteria for this study.

2. Identify the sample characteristics for this study.

3. What is the sample size? _____________ Was a power analysis done to determine sample size? _____________ If so, what were the specifics for the power analysis?

4. Was the sample size adequate? Provide a rationale.

5. What was the sample mortality for this study?

6. Was probability or nonprobability sampling used in this study?

____

7. What specific type of sampling method was used in this study?

____

8. Was the sample in this study representative of the population studied? Provide a rationale.

9. Can the findings be generalized? Provide a rationale.

chapter 9 Measurement and Data Collection in Research

INTRODUCTION

You need to read Chapter 9 and then complete the following exercises. These exercises will assist you in learning relevant terms and identifying and critiquing measurement and data collection procedures in published studies.

RELEVANT TERMS

Directions: Define the following terms in your own words without looking at your textbook. Then check your definitions with those in the glossary of your textbook. Using this strategy, you can identify elements of the term that are not yet clear in your mind. Reread that section of the chapter to clarify your understanding of the term.

Direct measurement ____

____

Indirect measurement ____

____

Instrumentation ____

____

Nominal-scale measurement ____

____

Ordinal-scale measurement ____

____

Interval-scale measurement ____

____

Measurement error ____

____

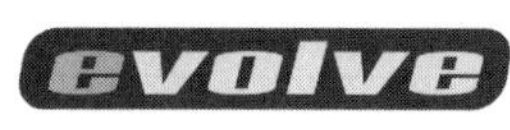

Be sure to check out the free exercises on-line at http://evolve.elsevier.com/Burns/understanding

Precision ____

____

Accuracy ____

____

Reliability ____

____

Validity ____

____

KEY IDEAS

Directions: Fill in the blanks with the appropriate word(s) or numbers.

1. The purpose of measurement is to produce ______________________ data.
2. The ideal, perfect measure is referred to as the ______________________ measure.
3. Measurement ______________________ is the difference between true measure and what, in reality, is measured.
4. Weight is an example of ______________________ measurement.
5. A coping scale is an example of ______________________ measurement.
6. A reliability value of ______________________ is considered the lowest acceptable coefficient for a well-developed measurement tool.

Random Error

Directions: Describe three situations that might result in random error.

1. ____
2. ____
3. ____

Systematic Error

Directions: Describe three measurement situations that might result in systematic error.

1. ____
2. ____
3. ____

Data Collection Tasks

Directions: List five tasks of the researcher during data collection

1. ______________________________
2. ______________________________
3. ______________________________
4. ______________________________
5. ______________________________

MAKING CONNECTIONS

Measurement Error

Directions: Match the type of measurement error likely to occur with the measurement method.

a. Random error
b. Systematic error

____ 1. Community income using a white, middle-class sample
____ 2. Severity of cancer at diagnosis in community using patients in a county hospital.
____ 3. Average body weight measured at work at noon.
____ 4. Blood pressure taken with a stethoscope from which it is difficult to hear.
____ 5. Scores on drug calculation test taken in clinical setting anytime during work shift.

Level of Measurement

Directions: Match the level of measurement with the measures listed below.

a. Nominal
b. Ordinal
c. Interval or higher

____ 1. Temperature
____ 2. Gender
____ 3. Educational level
____ 4. Final exam grade
____ 5. Type of cancer
____ 6. Severity of illness rank
____ 7. Score from visual analogue scale

Type of Reliability or Validity

Directions: Match the type of reliability or validity with the definition.

____ 1. Test-retest reliability
____ 2. Interrater reliability
____ 3. Homogeneity
____ 4. Content validity
____ 5. Validity evidence from contrasting groups
____ 6. Validity evidence from examining convergence
____ 7. Validity evidence from examining divergence
____ 8. Validity evidence from discriminant analysis
____ 9. Validity evidence from predicting future events
____ 10. Validity evidence from predicting concurrent events
____ 11. Accuracy
____ 12. Precision
____ 13. Sensitivity

a. Comparison of values with those of other instruments that measure the same concept
b. Amount of change that can be measured
c. Comparison of values with those of other instruments that measure similar concepts
d. Consistency of measurement of two raters
e. Comparison of groups expected to have opposing responses to instrument items
f. Adequacy of operational definition
g. Evaluates consistency of repeated measures
h. Comparison of values with those of other instruments that measure opposite concepts
i. Ability of instrument values to predict future performance
j. Ability to predict current value of measure based on value from measure of another concept
k. Correlation of various items within an instrument
l. consistency of measurement
m. Extent to which all elements of a concept are measured

EXERCISES IN CRITIQUE

Measuring Variables

Directions: Review the research articles in Appendix B and answer the following questions.

Using the following tables, identify the variables measured, the method of measurement, and the directness of measurement (D = direct, I = indirect).

Carey, Nicholson, and Fox study

Variable	Method of Measurement	Directness

Carey, Nicholson, and Fox study (cont'd)

Variable	Method of Measurement	Directness

Lewis et al. study

Variable	Method of Measurement	Directness

Bruce and Grove study

Variable	Method of Measurement	Directness

Describing Measures

Directions: Critique the thoroughness with which each method of measurement was described. In making this judgment, look for the following information about the measurement method:

1. Developer of the method of measurement
2. Date measurement method was developed
3. Detailed description of method of measurement (i.e., number of items in scale, steps of performing a physiologic measure)
4. Range of values possible using the measure

Carey et al. study

a. Measure ____

b. Measure ____

c. Measure ____

d. Measure ____

e. Measure ____

Lewis et al. study

a. Measure ______________________________

Bruce and Grove study

a. Measure ______________________________

b. Measure ____

c. Measure ____

d. Measure ____

Reliability and Validity of Measures

Directions: To examine the reliability and validity of each measure, identify the types of reliability and validity reported for each measure and the numerical values reported for each using the following table. Of particular interest is whether reliability was examined in the sample used in the study.

Carey et al. study

Measure ______________________________

Type of Reliability or Validity	Value	From present sample?

Measure ______________________________

Type of Reliability or Validity	Value	From present sample?

Measure ______________________________

Type of Reliability or Validity	Value	From present sample?

Measure ______________________________

Type of Reliability or Validity	Value	From present sample?

Measure ______________________________

Type of Reliability or Validity	Value	From present sample?

Lewis et al. study

Measure ______________________________

Type of Reliability or Validity	Value	From present sample?

Bruce and Grove study

Measure ______________________________

Type of Reliability or Validity	Value	From present sample?

Measure ______________________________

Type of Reliability or Validity	Value	From present sample?

Measure ____

Type of Reliability or Validity	Value	From present sample?

Measure ____

Type of Reliability or Validity	Value	From present sample?

Description of Data Collection

Directions: In each study, look for a description of the data collection process. Look for inconsistencies in measurements. Identify threats to the validity of the measures.

Carey et al. study

Lewis et al. study

Bruce and Grove study

Judging Measurement Adequacy

Directions: Using the information gathered in the previous exercise, judge the adequacy of each measure used in each study.

Carey et al. study

Lewis et al. study

Bruce and Grove study

GOING BEYOND

Identify a quasi-experimental study in a recent nursing journal. Identify the intervention or treatment. Was the intervention described in sufficient detail for you to provide the same intervention? Was the intervention provided consistently to all subjects? In your opinion, was the intervention sufficiently powerful to cause a difference in effect between the experimental and control groups? Write a brief paragraph judging the adequacy of the intervention.

chapter 10 Understanding Statistics in Research

INTRODUCTION

You need to read Chapter 10 and then complete the following exercises. These exercises will assist you in learning relevant terms and identifying and critiquing statistics or results sections in published studies.

RELEVANT TERMS

Directions: Define the following terms in your own words without looking at your textbook. Then check your definitions with those in the glossary of your textbook. Using this strategy, you can identify elements of the term that are not yet clear in your mind. Reread that section of the chapter to clarify your understanding of the term.

Central tendency ____

____

Clinical significance ____

____

Dependent groups ____

____

Variance ____

____

Distribution ____

____

Frequencies ____

____

Generalization ____

____

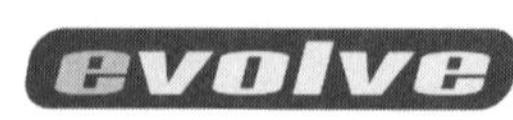

Be sure to check out the free exercises on-line at http://evolve.elsevier.com/Burns/understanding

Inference ____

____

Outliers ____

____

Power ____

____

Relationship ____

____

Statistic ____

____

Tailedness ____

____

List four activities of data cleaning.

1. ____
2. ____
3. ____
4. ____

List three statistical strategies used to describe the sample.

1. ____
2. ____
3. ____

MAKING CONNECTIONS

Directions: Perform the following matching exercises.

Matching Definitions

____ 1. Exploratory analysis
____ 2. Outliers
____ 3. Probability
____ 4. Inference
____ 5. Generalization
____ 6. Type I error
____ 7. Type II error
____ 8. Power
____ 9. Decision theory

a. Accepts null hypothesis when it is false
b. The probability that a statistical test will detect a significant difference that exists
c. Conclusion based on evidence
d. Information applied to a population that has been acquired from a specific instance
e. Rejects null hypothesis when it is true
f. The likelihood of an event occurring in a given situation
g. Assumption of no difference
h. Subjects with extreme values
i. Descriptive examination of the data

Matching Categories to Statements

a. Decision theory statement
b. Probability theory statement
c. Inference
d. Generalization

_____ 1. As hypothesized, the experimental systematic nursing assessment successfully forestalled the increase in symptom distress (Sarna, 1998, p. 1044).

_____ 2. This suggests that when psychological distress occurs, disruption in sexual activity and sexual desire also is likely to be present (Steginga, Occhipinti, Wilson, & Dunn, 1998, p. 1068).

_____ 3. No significant differences in functional and psychosocial outcomes were found between the two groups of patients treated with AMP [amputation] or LS [limb-sparing] surgical procedure (Hudson, Tyc, Cremer, Luo, Li, Rao, Meyer, Crom, & Pratt, 1998, p. 68).

_____ 4. Because most major risk factors thought to affect skin health did not change (i.e., body movement, skin moisture, fecal incontinence/frequency) and no adverse changes in skin health were observed during the intervention period, it is plausible to argue that the individualized intervention would not have adverse skin effects if applied over longer time periods (Schnelle, Criuse, Alessi, Al-Samarrai, & Ouslander, 1998, p. 203).

_____ 5. The results of this study indicate that GBI [geragogy-based instruction] can aid in increasing medication knowledge in a rural elderly ED [emergency department] population. Written medication instructions that are typed in large print, understandable on a fourth- to fifth-grade reading level, and organized in the elderly schema for remembering medications appear to be successful in the teaching and learning of medication information (Hayes, 1998, p. 216).

_____ 6. The results of the path analysis provided empirical support for the theoretical model of the direct and indirect effects of perceived self-efficacy on depressive symptoms (Kurlowicz, 1998, p. 223).

_____ 7. Automatic cuffs can be used safely for frequent assessment of blood pressure in patients with acute myocardial infarction who are receiving thrombolytic therapy (Saul, Smith, & Mook, 1998, p. 195).

Significant Differences

In testing for significant differences between groups, the researcher is determining whether the experimental group belongs to the same population as the control group. An initial step in this process is to compare the mean and standard deviation of the control group with those of the experimental group. The normal curve can be used to visually depict differences in these measures between the two groups. For example, Maloni, Chance, Zhang, Cohen, Betts, and Gange (1993) compared the physical and psychosocial side effects of antepartum hospital complete bed rest, partial bed rest, and no bed rest. Using the no-bed-rest group as the control group, we can compare these three groups. For the variable of weight gain, the no-bed-rest group mean (M) was 14.48 with a standard deviation (SD) of 4.94. Using this information, the distribution of weight gain in the no-bed-rest group can be illustrated.

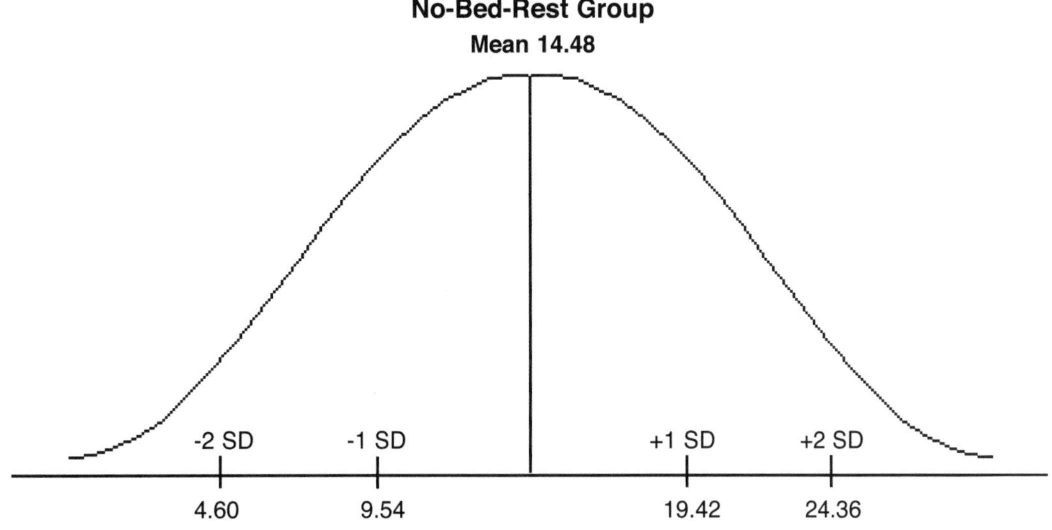

1. The mean for the partial-bed-rest group was 10.90 with a standard deviation of 5.29. Using the following curve, illustrate the distribution of values as shown on the previous page.

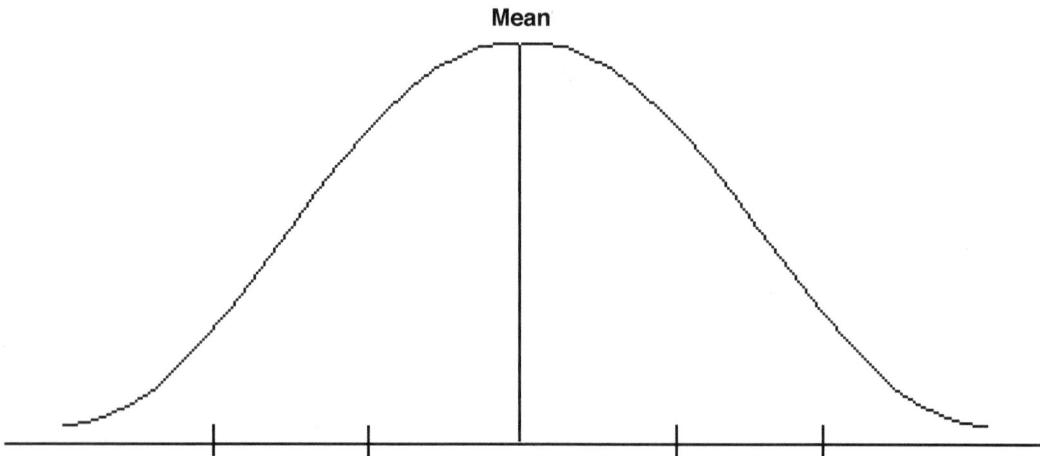

2. The mean for the complete-bed-rest group was 8.17 with a standard deviation of 2.09. Using the following curve, illustrate the distribution of values.

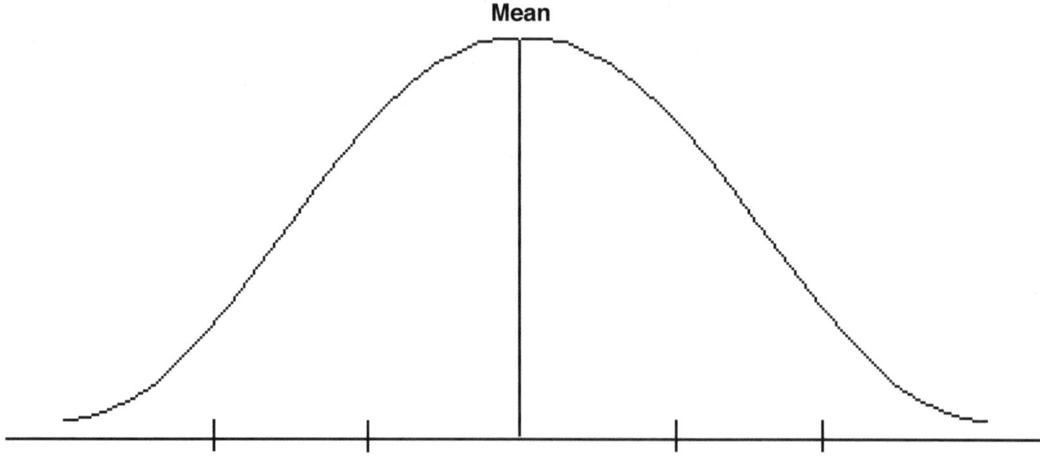

Statistical analyses are required to determine whether the differences in weight gain in the three groups indicates that the groups represent different populations. ANOVA results were $F = 7.79$ with df = 2,28 and $p = .002$, indicating that the groups are significantly different if alpha is set at .05.

Significance of Results

Directions: In the following statistical reports, indicate whether the results were significant, assuming a level of significance set at .05.

a. Significant
b. Not significant

_____ 1. The study examined psychosocial adjustment of males to three types of dialysis. ANOVA was used to examine differences among the three dialysis types. The results were as follows: $F = 4$, $p < .0467$ (Courts & Boyette, 1998, p. 54).

_____ 2. The study examined the safety of automatic versus manual blood pressure cuffs for patients receiving thrombolytic therapy. Purpura developed in 33 subjects (34%), 17 of whom had blood pressure measured with a manual cuff and 16 of whom had blood pressure measured with an automatic device ($p = .883$) (Saul, Smith & Mook, 1998).

_____ 3. The study examined the relationship between psychological distress and gastrointestinal symptoms in women with irritable bowel syndrome. There was a significant positive relationship between the Turmoil score [measuring psychological distress] and GI Distress score, $\beta = 0.47$, SE of $\beta = 0.11$, $t_{(96)} = 4.30$, $p < .001$ (Jarrett, Heitkempter, Cain, Tuftin, Walker, Bond, & Levy, 1998).

_____ 4. The study examined moderators of the relationship between trait anxiety and information received by patients postmyocardial infarction. When information received was regressed on the product of trait anxiety and gender, the beta was –.10 ($p = .42$) and the R^2 change was .009, $F = .66$, $p = .42$. (Yarcheski, Proctor, & Oriscello, 1998).

EXERCISES IN CRITIQUE

Directions: Refer to the Bruce and Grove study in Appendix B and answer the following questions. The research question for this study is: What is the difference in the mean total serum cholesterol, LDL cholesterol, and HDL cholesterol and cardiovascular risk levels of military members before and after participation in the C.A.R.E. program?

1. List the variables that will be used in statistical analyses to answer the Bruce and Grove research question and indicate the level of measurement of each variable.

Variable	Level of Measurement

2. Bruce and Grove chose to conduct two separate statistical analyses to answer their research questions, using the variables listed above. What were these statistical procedures?

   a.

   b.

3. Identify the groups used in the first analysis described in Bruce and Grove's research paper.

   a.

   b.

4. Were these two groups independent or dependent?

5. Using the algorithm in Chapter 10 of your textbook, judge the appropriateness of the statistical procedure used for the analysis. Can you identify other statistical procedures that might have been better? Write a brief paragraph expressing your judgment.

6. One variable was excluded from the first analysis. What was this variable?

7. Why was this variable excluded? (Use the information from question 1 in this section. In your textbook, reread the discussion on the statistical procedure selected for this analysis.)

8. State the results of the analysis, providing numerical values. Indicate whether each result is significant and predicted, nonsignificant, significant and not predicted, mixed result, or unexpected.

9. Identify the groups used in the second analysis described in Bruce and Grove's research paper.

   a.

   b.

10. Using the algorithm in Chapter 10 of your textbook, judge the appropriateness of the statistical procedure used for the analysis. Can you identify other statistical procedures that might have been better? Write a brief paragraph expressing your judgment.

11. State the results of the analysis, providing numerical values. Indicate whether the results are significant and predicted, nonsignificant, significant and not predicted, mixed results, or unexpected.

12. A third statistical procedure was performed that was not necessary to answer the research question but provided additional information about the variables. What was this procedure?

13. Identify the variables included in each of the three correlational analyses and the results. Indicate whether each result is significant and predicted, nonsignificant, significant and not predicted, mixed result, or unexpected.

    a.

    b.

    c.

14. Identify the findings reported by the authors. Compare these findings with the results you have just examined. Judge the appropriateness of the findings in relation to the results. Write a short paragraph below giving your evaluation of the linkage between the results and the findings.

15. Write a brief paragraph discussing the strengths and weakness of the analysis strategies used in the study.

16. Identify conclusions made by the authors based on their findings.

17. Write a brief paragraph judging whether the conclusions are warranted by the data.

18. Identify the implications made by the authors.

19. Write a brief paragraph evaluating these implications. Include implications you were able to identify that were not considered by the authors.

20. Write a brief paragraph assessing the clinical significance of these findings.

21. Were the findings generalized? If so, to what populations?

22. What suggestions did the authors make for further studies?

GOING BEYOND

Perform a similar critique of the analyses used by Carey, Nicholson, and Fox's study.

References

Courts, N. F., & Boyette, B. G. (1998). Psychosocial adjustment of males on three types of dialysis. *Clinical Nursing Research, 7*(1), 47-63.

Hayes, K. (1998). Randomized trial of geragogy-based medication instruction in the emergency department. *Nursing Research, 47*(4), 211-218.

Hudson, M. M., Tyc, V. L., Cremer, L. K., Luo, X., Rao, B. N., Meyer, W. H., Crom, D. B., & Pratt, C. B. (1998). Patient satisfaction after limb-sparing surgery and amputation for pediatric malignant bone tumors. *Journal of Pediatric Oncology Nursing, 15*(2), 60-69.

Kurlowicz, L. H. (1998). Perceived self-efficacy, functional ability, and depressive symptoms in older elective surgery patients. *Nursing Research, 47*(4), 219-226.

Sarna, L. (1998). Effectiveness of structured nursing assessment of symptom distress in advanced lung cancer. *Oncology Nursing Forum, 25*(6), 1041–1048.

Saul, L., Smith, J., & Mook, W. (1998). The safety of automatic versus manual blood pressure cuffs for patients receiving thrombolytic therapy. *American Journal of Critical Care, 7*(3), 192–196.

Schnelle, J. F., Criuse, P. A., Alessi, C. A., Al-Samarrai, N., & Ouslander, J. G. (1998). Individualizing nighttime incontinence care in nursing home residents. *Nursing Research, 47*(4), 197–204.

Stenginga, S., Occhipinti, S., Wilson, K., & Dunn, J. (1998). Domains of distress: The experience of breast cancer in Australia. *Oncology Nursing Forum, 25*(6), 1063–1070.

Yarcheski, A., Proctor, T. F., & Oriscello, R. G. (1998). Moderators of the relationship between trait anxiety and information received by patients post-myocardial infarction. *Clinical Nursing Research, 7*(1), 29–46.

Fawcett, J., Pollio, N., Tully, A., Barron, M., Henklein, J. C., & Jones, R. C. (1993). Effects of information on adaptation to cesarean birth. *Nursing Research, 42*(1), 49–53.

Griffith, P., James, B., & Cropp, A. (1994). Evaluation of the safety and efficacy of topical nitroglycerin ointment to facilitate venous cannulation. *Nursing Research, 43*(4), 203–206.

Maloni, J. A., Chance, B., Zhang, C., Cohen, A. W., Betts, D., & Gange, S. J. (1993). Physical and psychosocial side effects of antepartum hospital bed rest. *Nursing Research, 42*(4), 197–203.

Metheny, N., Reed, L., Wiersema, L., McSweeney, M., Wehrle, M. A., & Clark, J. (1993). Effectiveness of pH measurements in predicting feeding tube placement: An update. *Nursing Research, 42*(6), 324–331.

O'Brien, M. T. (1993). Multiple sclerosis: The relationship among self-esteem, social support, and coping behavior. *Applied Nursing Research, 6*(2), 54–63.

Shoaf, J., & Oliver, S. (1992). Efficacy of normal saline injection with and without heparin for maintaining intermittent intravenous site. *Applied Nursing Research, 5*(1), 9–12.

Wakefield, B., Wakefield, D. S., & Booth, B. M. (1992). Evaluating the validity of blood glucose monitoring strip interpretation by experienced users. *Applied Nursing Research, 5*(1), 13–19.

chapter 11 Introduction to Qualitative Research

INTRODUCTION

You need to read Chapter 11 and then complete the following exercises. These exercises will assist you in learning relevant terms and reading and comprehending published qualitative studies.

RELEVANT TERMS

Directions: Define the following terms in your own words without looking at your textbook. Then check your definitions with those in the glossary of your textbook. Using this strategy, you can identify elements of the term that are not yet clear in your mind. Reread that section of the chapter to clarify your understanding of the term.

Decision trail ____

____

Holistic ____

____

Reductionism ____

____

Reflexive thought ____

____

Rigor ____

____

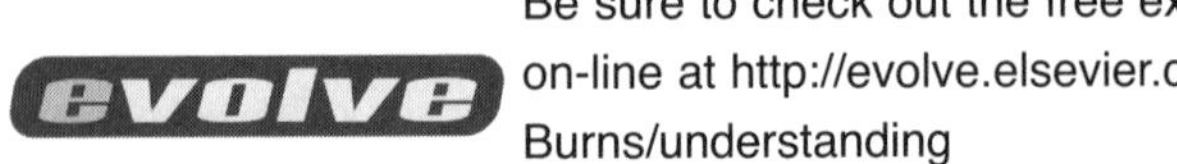

MAKING CONNECTIONS

Directions: Match each type of research with its characteristics.

a. Qualitative
b. Quantitative

____ 1. Produced "hard" science
____ 2. Philosophical approach to research
____ 3. Truth is absolute
____ 4. Reductionistic
____ 5. Holistic
____ 6. Researcher remains objective and detached
____ 7. Truth is dynamic
____ 8. Control is important
____ 9. Subjectivity is essential
____ 10. Unstructured

Directions: List three characteristics of rigor in qualitative studies.

1. ______________________________
2. ______________________________
3. ______________________________

Directions: List three characteristics of researcher-participant relationships in qualitative research.

1. ______________________________
2. ______________________________
3. ______________________________

Directions: List four methods of reducing data in qualitative research.

1. ______________________________
2. ______________________________
3. ______________________________
4. ______________________________

Directions: List three methods of drawing conclusions commonly used in qualitative studies.

1. ______________________________
2. ______________________________
3. ______________________________

Directions: Match each qualitative method with its characteristics.

a. Phenomenological
b. Grounded theory
c. Ethnographic
d. Historical

____ 1. Studies cultures
____ 2. Studies interactions of individuals or groups
____ 3. Studies meaning of a lived experience
____ 4. Uses informants
____ 5. Used by Benner to examine clinical practice
____ 6. Studies the past
____ 7. Gaining entry is essential
____ 8. Uses constant comparative process
____ 9. Develops an inventory of sources
____ 10. Considers an experience unique to the individual

Directions: List three stages of qualitative data analysis.

1. ______________________________
2. ______________________________
3. ______________________________

Storytelling

Directions: Tape-record a story told to you by a friend or family member. Write the story in narrative form, in steps, using the following categories:

1. What is this about?
2. Who? What? When? Where?
3. Then what happened?
4. So what?
5. What finally happened?
6. Finish narrative

What is the purpose of the story?

1. Make a point
2. Be moralistic
3. A success story
4. A reminder of what not to do or how not to be
5. Guidance in how to avoid the fate described in the story

EXERCISES IN CRITIQUE

Directions: Examine the qualitative component in the Carey, Nicholson, and Fox study.

1. What approach did the authors use to analyze the qualitative data?

2. Identify the themes that emerged from the analysis.

3. How did the authors validate the identified themes?

4. Read the discussion of qualitative findings in the discussion section. How did the authors compare quantitative and qualitative findings?

5. In the implications section under Active Listening, the implications of the qualitative findings are discussed. What do the authors recommend?

GOING BEYOND

Select a qualitative study from a recent nursing journal and complete the following.

1. Identify the type of qualitative study performed.
2. Identify the data collection methods used.
3. What were the relationships between the researcher and participants?
4. Identify the following steps of data analysis:
   a. Description
   b. Analysis
   c. Interpretation
5. Evaluate the rigor of the study.
6. Do the authors address a decision trail?

chapter 12 Critiquing Nursing Studies

INTRODUCTION

You need to read Chapter 12 and then complete the following exercises. These exercises will assist you in understanding the quantitative and qualitative research critique processes. The answers to these exercises are in Appendix A under Chapter 12.

RELEVANT TERMS

Directions: Match each term with its correct definition.

a. Analysis step of critique
b. Analytic preciseness
c. Auditability
d. Comparison step of critique
e. Comprehension step of critique
f. Descriptive vividness
g. Evaluation step of critique
h. Heuristic relevance
i. Methodological congruence
j. Theoretical connectedness

Definitions

_____ 1. Standard for evaluating qualitative research, in which documentation rigor, procedural rigor, ethical rigor, and auditability of the study are examined.

_____ 2. Rigorous development of a decision trail that is reported in sufficient detail to allow a second researcher to use the original data and the decision trail to arrive at conclusions similar to those of the original researcher.

_____ 3. Critique step that involves determining the strengths and limitations of the logical links connecting one study element with another.

_____ 4. Theoretical schema developed from a qualitative study; is clearly expressed, logically consistent, reflective of the data, and compatible with nursing's knowledge base.

_____ 5. Critique step in which the reader examines the meaning and significance of a study according to set criteria and compares it with previous studies conducted in the area.

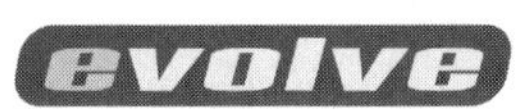

Be sure to check out the free exercises on-line at http://evolve.elsevier.com/Burns/understanding

_____ 6. Performing a series of transformations during which concrete data are transformed across several levels of abstractions to develop a theoretical schema that imparts meaning to the phenomenon under study.

_____ 7. Critique step during which the reader gains understanding of the terms in the research report; identifies the study elements and grasps the nature, significance, and meaning of these elements.

_____ 8. Standard for evaluating a qualitative study, in which the study's intuitive recognition, relationship to the existing body of knowledge, and applicability are examined.

_____ 9. Description of the site, subjects, experience of collecting data, and the researcher's thoughts during the qualitative research process; presented clearly enough that the reader has the sense of personally experiencing the event.

_____ 10. Critique step in which the ideal for each step of the quantitative research process is compared with the real steps in a published study.

KEY IDEAS

Directions: Fill in the blanks with the appropriate word(s).

1. An intellectual research critique involves careful examination of all aspects of a study to judge the ____________________, ____________________, ____________________, and ____________________ of the study.
2. Identify three important questions that are part of an intellectual research critique.
   a. ____
   b. ____
   c. ____
3. Describe your role in conducting research critiques.
4. List the four steps of the quantitative research critique process.
   a. ____________________ c. ____________________
   b. ____________________ d. ____________________

5. Identify the five standards used to critique qualitative studies.

   a. ______________________________

   b. ______________________________

   c. ______________________________

   d. ______________________________

   e. ______________________________

EXERCISES IN CRITIQUE

Directions: Read the research articles in Appendix B. Conduct the different steps of the quantitative research critique process (comprehension, comparison, analysis, and evaluation) on these three studies using the guidelines in Chapter 12, Critiquing Nursing Studies, in your textbook.

1. Conduct a critique of the Carey, Nicholson, and Fox (2002) article using the guidelines outlined in your text. Many parts of this study were critiqued in Chapters 3–10 of this study guide.

   a. Conduct the comprehension step of the critique process. Questions are outlined in your text to direct your critique.

   b. Do a critique that includes the comparison, analysis, and evaluation steps of the quantitative research critique process.

2. Conduct a critique of the Lewis, P., Nichols, E., Mackey, G., Fadol, A., Sloane, L., Villagomez, E., and Liehr, P. (1997) article using the guidelines outlined in your text. Many parts of this study were critiqued in Chapters 3–10 of this study guide.

   a. Conduct the comprehension step of the critique process. Questions are outlined in your text to direct your critique.

   b. Do a critique that includes the comparison, analysis, and evaluation steps of the quantitative research critique process.

3. Conduct a critique of the Bruce and Grove (1994) article using the guidelines outlined in your text. Many parts of this study were critiqued in Chapters 3–10 of this study guide.

   a. Conduct the comprehension step of the critique process. Questions are outlined in your text to direct your critique.

   b. Do a critique that includes the comparison, analysis, and evaluation steps of the quantitative research critique process.

chapter 13 Using Research in Nursing Practice with a Goal of Evidence-Based Practice

INTRODUCTION

You need to read Chapter 13 and then complete the following exercises. These exercises will assist you in understanding the process for using research findings in practice. The answers to these exercises are in Appendix A under Chapter 13.

RELEVANT TERMS

Directions: Match each term with its definition or description.

a. Communication of research findings
b. Conduct and Utilization of Research in Nursing (CURN) Project
c. Innovation
d. Innovators
e. Meta-analysis
f. Research utilization
g. Rogers' Innovation-Decision Process
h. Western Interstate Commission for Higher Education (WICHE) regional nursing research development project

Definitions

_____ 1. The use of statistical analysis and the interpretations of the results to merge the findings from several studies to determine what is known about a particular phenomenon.
_____ 2. Process that includes the steps of knowledge, persuasion, decision, implementation, and confirmation to promote diffusion or communication of research findings to members of a discipline.
_____ 3. Process by which research knowledge is communicated to members of a social system to achieve a desired outcome.
_____ 4. Developing a research report and disseminating it through presentations and publications to practicing nurses, other health professionals, consumers, and policy makers.

_____ 5. Idea, practice, or object that is perceived as new by an individual, a nursing unit, an entire agency, or other decision-making unit.

_____ 6. First major research utilization project in nursing that involved the collaboration of clinicians and educators in critiquing studies and developing detailed plans for using selected research findings in practice.

_____ 7. Individuals who actively seek out new ideas.

_____ 8. Project in which the purpose was to increase the use of research findings in practice by communicating the findings, facilitating organizational modifications necessary for implementation, and encouraging collaborative research that is directly useful in clinical practice.

KEY IDEAS

Directions: Fill in the blanks with the appropriate word(s).

1. List four reasons why nurses need to use research findings in practice.

   a. ______________________________

   b. ______________________________

   c. ______________________________

   d. ______________________________

2. Think about the clinical agency where you are currently doing your clinical hours.

   a. Are the agency's policies and nursing protocols based on research?

   b. If you answered "no" to the previous question, what is the basis of the policies and protocols of your agency?

   c. Who are the innovators in this agency? (Just record the persons' positions.)

d. Who might be resistant to change?

e. Does the agency provide research publications for nurses? If so, provide some examples of these publications.

3. Identify three sources that you might access to keep current with the research literature.

   a. ______________________________

   b. ______________________________

   c. ______________________________

4. Identify two reports that were published from the WICHE project.

   a. ______________________________

   b. ______________________________

5. Identify the four-step research utilization process used in the CURN project.

   a. ______________________________

   b. ______________________________

   c. ______________________________

   d. ______________________________

6. Identify six topics for which research findings were considered worthy of implementation in practice in the CURN project.

   a. ______________________________

   b. ______________________________

   c. ______________________________

   d. ______________________________

   e. ______________________________

   f. ______________________________

7. Identify the three types of barriers to using research findings in nursing practice. Provide an example of each.

   a. ______________________________

      Example ______________________________

   b. ______________________________

      Example ______________________________

   c. ______________________________

      Example ______________________________

8. Identify three prior conditions of an agency that need to be examined when planning to make a change based on research.

   a. ______________________________

   b. ______________________________

   c. ______________________________

9. Identify the five characteristics of the innovation or change in practice that need to be examined during the persuasion stage.

   a. ______________________________

   b. ______________________________

   c. ______________________________

   d. ______________________________

   e. ______________________________

10. Active rejection of a change in practice involves ______________________________

    ______________________________.

11. Passive rejection of a change in practice indicates ______________________________

    ______________________________.

12. Identify and describe the three ways that research findings might be implemented in nursing practice.

    a. ____________________ Description ______________________________

    ____

b. ______________________ Description ______________________

____

c. ______________________ Description ______________________

____

13. During the confirmation stage, discontinuance of the change in practice can occur. What are the two types of discontinuance?

 a. ____

 b. ____

14. Identify two sources of summaries of nursing research knowledge.

 a. ____

 b. ____

15. Evidenced-based practice is the careful and practical use of ______________ ______________________ evidence to guide health-care decisions.

16. Current best evidence includes clinical practice guidelines that are usually nationally developed by expert ______________, ______________, and ______________ in their areas of excellence.

17. Grove's algorithm for facilitating evidence-based practice in nursing identified three sources of evidence that might be used in your practice. What are these?

 a. ____

 b. ____

 c. ____

18. The ultimate goal of nursing is ______________-__________ practice.

19. A benchmark is an ____

____.

20. A research-based protocol provides ____

____.

21. Identify two Web sites that have nationally developed clinical practice guidelines.

    a. ______________________________

    b. ______________________________

MAKING CONNECTIONS

Directions: Match each stage in Rogers' Research Utilization Model with its appropriate description.

Stages

a. Knowledge
b. Persuasion
c. Decision
d. Implementation
e. Confirmation

Descriptions

_____ 1. The stage where the nurses evaluate the effectiveness of the change in practice and decide to either continue or discontinue it.

_____ 2. The stage where the innovation is either adopted or rejected.

_____ 3. The first awareness of the existence of an innovation or new idea for use in practice.

_____ 4. The stage where the innovation or change is put to use by an individual, unit, or agency.

_____ 5. The stage where an individual or agency develops a favorable or unfavorable attitude toward the change or innovation.

GOING BEYOND

Conduct a project to use research findings in practice. Use the content and example of research utilization in Chapter 13 and the following steps as a guide.

1. Identify a clinical problem that might be improved by using research knowledge.

2. Locate and review the studies in this problem area.

3. Summarize what is known and not known regarding this problem. (See Chapter 4 for additional direction in summarizing research literature).

4. Select a model or theory to direct your use of research findings in practice, such as Rogers' Research Utilization Model.

5. Assess your agency's readiness to make the change (prior conditions in Rogers' Model).

6. Persuade the nursing personnel, other health professionals, and administration to make the change in practice. (This is the persuasion stage of Rogers' Model.)

7. Have those persons involved in the change make a decision to adopt or reject the change (Rogers' decision stage).

8. Implement the change by developing a protocol or policy that will clearly indicate the change needed in practice. Communicate this protocol or policy to members of the clinical agency (Rogers' implementation stage).

9. Develop evaluation strategies to determine the effect of the change. You might examine cost, patient outcomes, and nursing workload (Rogers' confirmation stage).

10. Evaluate over time to determine whether the change continued. You might also extend the change to additional units or clinical agencies.

appendix A Answers to Study Guide Exercises

CHAPTER 1—DISCOVERING NURSING RESEARCH

Relevant Terms

1. f
2. g
3. a
4. d
5. i
6. l
7. b
8. o
9. e
10. n
11. k
12. c
13. h
14. m
15. j
16. p

Key Ideas

1. Description involves identifying the nature and attributes of nursing phenomena. Descriptive knowledge generated through research can be used to identify what exists in nursing practice, to discover new information, and to classify information of use in the discipline. For example, describing those who are at risk for HIV or identifying the signs and symptoms for making a nursing diagnosis.
2. Explanation focuses on clarifying relationships among variables or identifying reasons why certain events occur. For example, risk for developing pressure ulcers is related to level of mobility and age; as mobility decreases and age increases, pressure ulcer risk increases.
3. Prediction involves estimating the probability of a specific outcome in a given situation. With predictive knowledge, nurses could anticipate the effects nursing interventions would have on patients and families. For example, predicting the effects of a long-term exercise program on women with breast cancer.
4. Control is the ability to manipulate a situation to produce the desired outcome. Thus, nurses could prescribe certain interventions to help patients and families achieve quality outcomes. For example, you would prescribe the use of warm, not cold, applications for the resolution of normal saline IV infiltrations.

Historical Events Influencing Nursing Research

1. Nightingale
2. 1952
3. ANA Council of Nurse Researchers
4. research
5. *Research in Nursing & Health*
6. *Western Journal of Nursing Research*
7. *Scholarly Inquiry for Nursing Practice*
   Applied Nursing Research
   Nursing Science Quarterly
8. Conduct and Utilization of Research in Nursing (CURN)
9. integrative reviews of research or summaries of current research knowledge in the areas of nursing practice, nursing care delivery, nursing education, and the nursing profession
10. 1985
11. National Institute for Nursing Research (NINR)
12. conduct, support, and dissemination of information
13. The mission for NINR for the 21st Century is to "support clinical and basic research to establish a scientific basis for the care of individuals across the life-span—from management of patients during illness and recovery to the reduction of risks for disease and disability, the promotion of healthy lifestyles, promoting quality of life in those with chronic illness, and care for the individuals at the end of life" (search the NINR website: http://www.nih/gov/ninr).
14. clinical
15. Agency for Health Care Policy and Research (AHCPR)
16. scientific or empirical
17. Agency for Healthcare Research and Quality (AHRQ)
18. Evidence-based practice facilitates (a) promoting an understanding of patients' and families' experiences with health and illness; (b) implementing effective nursing interventions to promote patient health; and (c) providing quality, cost-effective care within the health care system.
19. *Healthy People 2010*
20. outcomes research

Acquiring Knowledge in Nursing

1. You could have identified any of the following ways of acquiring knowledge in nursing. Some possible examples of each way of acquiring nursing knowledge are provided.
   a. Tradition: giving report on hospitalized patients in a specific way or organizing the care provided to the patients in a specific, structured way.

- b. Authority: expert nurses, educators, and authors of articles or books
- c. Borrowing: using knowledge from medicine or psychology in nursing practice
- d. Trial and error: positioning a patient to reduce his or her discomfort
- e. Personal experience: obtaining knowledge by being in a clinical agency and providing care to patients and families
- f. Role-modeling: a new graduate in an internship being mentored by an expert nurse
- g. Intuition: knowing that a patient's condition is deteriorating but having no concrete data to support this feeling or hunch
- h. Reasoning: reasoning from the general to the specific or deductive reasoning; reasoning from the specific to the general or inductive reasoning.
- i. Research: quantitative, qualitative, and outcomes research methods

2. personal experience
3. novice, advanced beginner, competent, proficient, and expert
4. borrowed
5. research, empirical, or scientific
6. intuition
7. traditions
8. mentorship relationship
9. role-model
10. inductive and deductive
11. deductive reasoning
12. quantitative, qualitative, and outcomes
13. outcomes research
14. Identify common interventions used in practice, such as taking a temperature, providing oral care, treating an ulcer, changing a dressing on a wound. Use the content in your textbook on Acquiring Knowledge in Nursing to determine the knowledge base for each of the interventions you identified. Nursing knowledge is acquired through tradition, authority, borrowing, trial and error, personal experience, role-modeling, intuition, reasoning, and research.
15. You need to examine the interventions you use in clinical practice and decide which way of acquiring knowledge you use most frequently: tradition, authority, borrowing, trial and error, personal experience, role-modeling, intuition, reasoning, and research.
16. Important outcomes include outcomes such as patient health status (signs, symptoms, functional status, morbidity, mortality), patient satisfaction, costs related to health care, quality of care, quality of care provider, provider satisfaction, access to care by patients and families.

Making Connections

Types of Research Methods

1. b
2. b
3. a
4. b
5. a
6. a
7. a
8. b

Nurses' Educational Preparation

1. a
2. e
3. b
4. d
5. b
6. c
7. d

Puzzles

Quantitative, qualitative, and outcomes research are essential to develop evidence-based nursing practice.

Research knowledge is needed to control outcomes in nursing practice.

Exercises in Critique

Research Methods

1. b and c
2. c
3. c

Researchers' Credentials

1. Carey, Nicholson, and Fox all have PhD degrees, which indicates a background in the conduct of research. Both Fox and Nicholson have previously published parenting studies that are cited in the reference list. Carey conducted this study for her doctoral dissertation and received funding from the Children's Hospital Foundation, Milwaukee, WI. These individuals have very strong research preparation for conducting this study in addition to the funding. The clinical expertise of these individuals is unclear. No employment status was identified for the three authors.

2. Liehr is PhD-prepared and employed by the University of Texas Health Science Center in Houston. Lewis, Mackey, Fadol, Sloane, and Villagomez have master's degrees and are practicing in a variety of clinical facilities. Nichols has a BSN and was collaborating with others in this research project. These individuals appear to have strong research and clinical expertise to conduct this study.

3. Bruce is a master's (MSN)–prepared nurse who is providing care to individuals who have a history of hyperlipidemia and coronary artery disease. Grove is doctorally (PhD) prepared in nursing and has co-authored two nursing research textbooks. The military provided Bruce support for this project that was conducted with military personnel as the research subjects. These authors have strong educational preparation and clinical expertise to collaborate on a research project.

CHAPTER 2—INTRODUCTION TO THE QUANTITATIVE RESEARCH PROCESS

Relevant Terms

1. n
2. s
3. b
4. e
5. r
6. d
7. k
8. q
9. h
10. l
11. m
12. c
13. t
14. a
15. o
16. p
17. j
18. i
19. g
20. f

Key Ideas

Control in Quantitative Research

1. highly controlled
2. quasi-experimental and experimental
3. descriptive or correlational
4. experimental
5. nonrandom, random
6. natural
7. highly controlled
8. experimental
9. partially controlled
10. quasi-experimental

Steps of the Research Process

1. problem-solving and the nursing processes
2. problem and purpose
3. methodology
4. evaluation and revision
   outcomes, communication of findings, and use of findings in practice
5. Step 1: Research problem and purpose
   Step 2: Literature review
   Step 3: Study framework
   Step 4: Research objectives, questions, or hypotheses
   Step 5: Study variables
   Step 6: Assumptions
   Step 7: Limitations
   Step 8: Research design
   Step 9: Population and sample
   Step 10: Methods of Measurement
   Step 11: Data collection
   Step 12: Data analysis
   Step 13: Research outcomes, communication of findings, and use of findings in practice
6. Assumptions are statements taken for granted or considered true, even though they have not been scientifically tested.
7. You could identify any of the following assumptions.
   a. "People want to assume control of their own health problems.
   b. Stress should be avoided.
   c. People are aware of the experiences that most affect their life choices.
   d. Health is a priority for most people.
   e. People in underserved areas feel underserved.
   f. Most measurable attitudes are held strongly enough to direct behavior.
   g. Health professionals view health care in a different manner than do lay persons.
   h. Human biological and chemical factors show less variation than do cultural and social factors.
   i. The nursing process is the best way of conceptualizing nursing practice.
   j. Statistically significant differences relate to the variable or variables under consideration.
   k. People operate on the basis of cognitive information.
   l. Increased knowledge about an event lowers anxiety about the event.
   m. Receipt of health care at home is preferable to receipt of care in an institution." (Williams, M. A. (1980) Editorial: Assumptions in research. *Research in Nursing & Health*, *3*(2), p. 48.)

8. theoretical and methodological
9. Answer can include methodological or theoretical limitations. The methodological limitations include such factors as nonrepresentative sample, small sample size, weak designs, single setting, instruments with limited reliability and validity, limited control over data collection, weak implementation of the treatment, and improper use of statistical analyses. Theoretical limitations include weak definitions of concepts in framework, weak conceptual definitions of variables, poorly developed study framework, or unclear link between study variables and framework concepts.
10. A pilot study is a smaller version of a proposed study conducted to develop and/or refine the methodology, such as the treatment, instruments, or data collection process to be used in the larger study.
11. You could identify any of the following reasons for conducting a pilot study.
    a. To determine whether the proposed study is feasible (e.g., Are the subjects available? Does the researcher have the time and money to conduct the study?).
    b. To develop or refine a research treatment.
    c. To develop a protocol for the implementation of a treatment.
    d. To identify problems with the design.
    e. To determine whether the sample is representative of the population or whether the sampling technique is effective.
    f. To examine the reliability and validity of the research instruments.
    g. To develop or refine data collection instruments.
    h. To refine the data collection and analysis plan.
    i. To give the researcher experience with the subjects, setting, methodology, and methods of measurement.
    j. To try out data analysis techniques.

Reading Research Reports

1. You could identify any three of the following research journals.
    a. *Advances in Nursing Science*
    b. *Applied Nursing Research*
    c. *Clinical Nursing Research: An International Journal*
    d. *Journal of Nursing Scholarship*
    e. *Nursing Research*
    f. *Research in Nursing & Health*
    g. *Scholarly Inquiry for Nursing Practice: An International Journal*
    h. *Western Journal of Nursing Research*
2. You could identify any three of the following journals. A complete list of the journals in which research reports compose 50% or more of the journal content is provided in Table 2-3 of Chapter 2.
    a. *Issues in Comprehensive Pediatric Nursing*
    b. *Journal of Transcultural Nursing*

   c. *Heart & Lung: Journal of Critical Care*
   d. *Journal of Nursing Education*
   e. *Birth*
   f. *Nursing Diagnosis*
   g. *Public Health Nursing*
   h. *The Diabetes Educator*
   i. *Maternal-Child Nursing Journal*
   j. *Journal of Nursing Education*
3. introduction, methods, results, and discussion
4. design, sample, setting, methods of measurement, and data collection process
5. major findings, limitations of the study, conclusions drawn from the findings, implications of the findings for nursing, and recommendations for further research
6. introduction section
7. theories and studies
8. skimming, comprehending, and analyzing
9. comprehending
10. analyzing

Making Connections

Types of Quantitative Research

1. c
2. a
3. b
4. a
5. c
6. d
7. a
8. b
9. c
10. d
11. b
12. a
13. c
14. a
15. c
16. a
17. b
18. a
19. a
20. b

Puzzles

Word Scramble

Quantitative research methods include descriptive, correlational, quasi-experimental, and experimental studies.

Rigor and control are important in quantitative research.

Crossword Puzzle

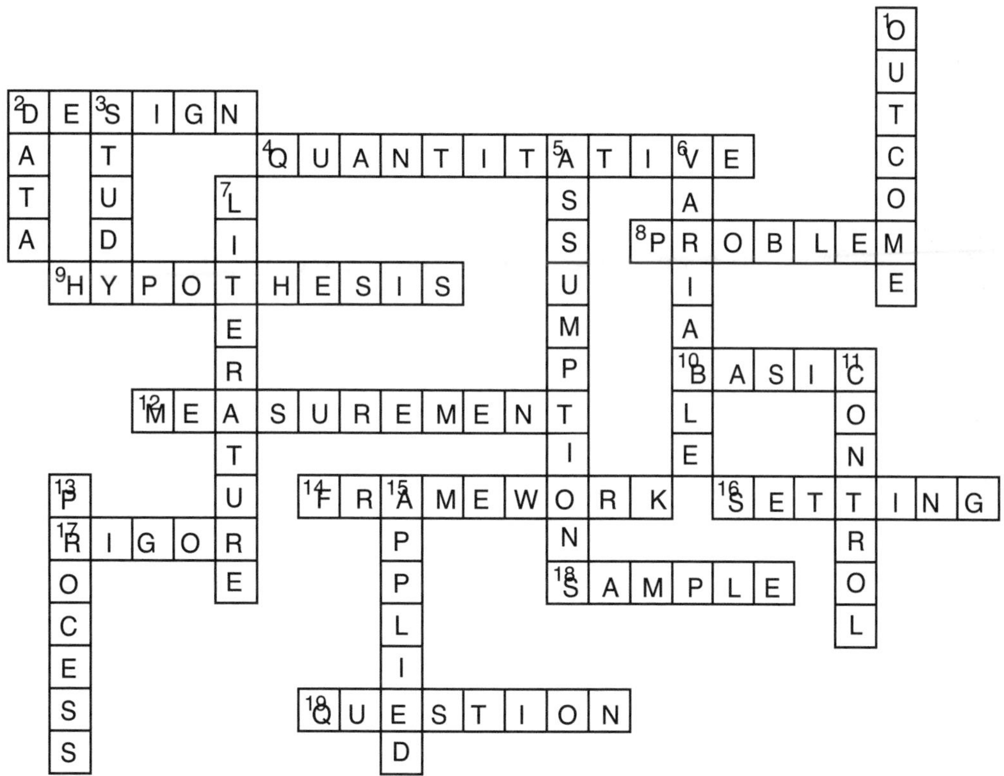

Exercises in Critique

Type of Quantitative Research

1. a Carey et al. (2002) has both a descriptive quantitative focus and an exploratory or qualitative focus.
2. c
3. a

Type of Setting

4. a Natural setting: Subjects' homes
5. b Partially controlled setting: Surgical intensive care unit (ICU) of a large urban hospital
6. b Partially controlled setting: Outpatient primary care clinical of a military hospital

Type of Research Conducted (Applied or Basic)

7. a
8. a
9. a

CHAPTER 3—RESEARCH PROBLEMS, PURPOSES, AND HYPOTHESES

Relevant Terms

Chapter Terms

1. f
2. i
3. h
4. g
5. j
6. k
7. e
8. d
9. a
10. c
11. b

Types of Hypotheses

1. h
2. g
3. b
4. e
5. c
6. a
7. d
8. f

Variables and Relevant Terms

1. a
2. d
3. f
4. c
5. e
6. b

Key Ideas

Research Problem and Purpose

1. variables, population, and setting
2. a. has an impact on nursing practice
   b. builds on previous research
   c. promotes theory development
   d. addresses current concerns or priorities in nursing.

3. You can identify any of the following agencies or organizations: National Institute for Nursing Research (NINR), American Association of Critical-Care Nurses (AACN), American Association of Occupational Health Nurses (AAOHN), Oncology Nursing Society (ONS), American Organization of Nurse Executives (AONE), or Agency for Healthcare Research and Quality (AHRQ).
4. a. researchers' expertise
   b. financial commitment
   c. availability of subjects, facility, and equipment
   d. study's ethical considerations
5. educational, clinical
6. objectives, questions, and hypotheses

Exercises in Critique

Carey et al. (2002) Study

1. "There are numerous factors that influence the quality of parenting that children receive (Belsky, 1990). The health status of a child, including the onset of a chronic illness, is one of many factors that can contribute to the quality of child rearing (Kazak, 1989). When considering that up to 30% of children have a chronic health condition (Newacheck & Halfon, 1998), 11% of whom are living with conditions considered moderate to severe (Newacheck, Stoddard, & McManus, 1993), a significant number of families are faced with an even more challenging future than they had anticipated. How parents respond to this situation can affect both the short- and long-term developmental outcomes for their children" (p. 198).
   "Most available studies regarding the parenting of children with CHD have emphasized parental adjustment to diagnosis (Emery, 1989), the demands and related stress that these children place on the family (Svavarstottir & McCubbin, 1996), and early care-giving issues, particularly infant feeding difficulties (Lobo, 1992). Relatively less attention has been devoted to the emotional adjustment of these children . . ." (p. 200).
2. "The purpose of this study was to compare the early child-rearing practices between mothers of children with congenital heart disease (CHD) and mothers of healthy children. In addition, parenting stress, parental expectations of their young children, and the early behavioral and emotional development of toddlers and preschoolers were explored" (p. 199).
3. The problem and purpose of the Carey et al. (2002) study are significant. The problem and purpose provide the basis for conducting a comparative descriptive quantitative study with an exploratory or qualitative part that focused on parenting responses. This exploratory descriptive study adds to our understanding of parenting responses of mothers of healthy children and of mothers of children with a chronic disease, CHD. This is an applied study with findings that have direct implications for nursing practice that are detailed by the authors in the

discussion section of the study. The study is soundly based on previous research and theory that is documented in the framework and literature review sections of this article. This is a significant study because 30% of the children have chronic health conditions and 11% of those have moderate to severe conditions. Additional research is essential to expand our understanding of the parenting process for children with chronic disease, to identify the factors that contribute to positive parenting behaviors, and to test the effectiveness of nursing interventions to facilitate positive parenting.

4. Variables: Child-rearing practices, parenting stress, parental expectations of young children, and early behavioral and emotional development
   Population: Mothers with young healthy children and mothers of young children with CHD.
   Setting: Subjects' homes in an urban area
5. The study has a feasible purpose. The authors had strong research expertise, developed an ethical study, identified appropriate measurement methods, and had adequate equipment to conduct the study. This study "was supported in part by a grant from the Children's Hospital Foundation, Milwaukee, WI" (p. 182). A weakness of the study was the small sample size for the quantitative descriptive aspect of this study.

Lewis et al. Study

1. "Backrubs and changes in body position are established interventions for enhancing patients' comfort, mobilizing pulmonary secretions, and improving tissue perfusion through pressure reduction. Understanding the best strategies for combining these interventions may improve patients' outcomes and make the best use of nursing time.
   Patients are commonly repositioned to the supine, right lateral, and left lateral positions before a backrub. The physiological effect of these interventions is questioned only if untoward changes are noted. Vital signs are routinely used to assess patients' responses to interventions such as changes in position and backrubs. Another useful measurement is mixed venous oxygen saturation (SvO_2), an indicator of oxygen delivery and consumption.
   Normally, patients are given a backrub immediately after a change in body position. The consequences of multiple, sequential activities can be hemodynamic compromise. We were interested in comparing the effects on SvO_2 of turning with immediate backrub and turning with a delayed backrub" (p. 218). This problem is expressed in the first few paragraphs of the article.
2. The purpose of this study was "to examine the effect of a change in body position (right or left lateral) and timing of backrub (immediate or delayed) on mixed venous oxygen saturation in surgical ICU patients" (p. 217).

3. The problem and purpose are significant and provide a basis for the generation of research questions that guide the remaining steps of the study. The study focuses on nursing interventions (backrub and positioning) and produces significant findings that can be used in the care of ICU patients. The importance of this research is to determine how to maximize nursing interventions to optimize oxygenation and prevent an imbalance between oxygen supply and demand in the ICU patient.
4. Variables: Body position (right or left lateral), timing of backrub (immediate or delayed), and mixed venous oxygen saturation
   Population: Surgical ICU patients
   Setting: Surgical ICU in large urban hospital
5. The authors have strong educational preparation and clinical expertise and have conducted and published previous research in this area. The authors had access to an adequate, critically ill, male patient population at the Veterans Affairs Medical Center, Houston, Texas. The study was ethical and required limited equipment since the pulmonary artery catheters were already in place for the measurement of SvO_2. The treatments of positioning and backrub were within the practice realm of the nurse.

Bruce and Grove Study

1. "Cardiovascular diseases cause nearly one of every two deaths in adults 45 years and older . . . It ranks first in terms of social security disability and second only to all forms of arthritis for limitation of activity, and to all forms of cancer combined for total hospital stays. In direct health care costs, lost wages, and productivity, coronary artery disease (CAD) costs the United States more than $60 billion a year . . . Risk factors for CAD include male gender, family history of premature CAD, diabetes mellitus, hypertension, high cholesterol, cigarette smoking, and obesity . . . Education can promote changes in daily living that reduce the risk for CAD . . . The goal of all risk-factor reduction strategies is to change blood lipid profiles from a 'bad' one (high LDL, low HDL) to a 'good' one (low LDL, high HDL)" (Bruce & Grove, 1994, pp. 231-232). This study problem was clearly stated in the first paragraph of the article.
2. "The purpose of this study was to compare a military population's mean levels of total serum cholesterol, LDL, HDL, and risk for cardiovascular disease (based on serum lipid levels) before and six months after a coronary artery risk evaluation (C.A.R.E.) program" (Bruce & Grove, 1994, p. 232).
3. The problem is significant to nursing because the C.A.R.E. program could be implemented by nurses in practice to improve the outcomes for patients with CAD. This could decrease the cost of health care and increase the patients' quality of life. This study builds on a solid base of previous research.
4. a. Variables: C.A.R.E. program, LDL, HDL, total serum cholesterol, and risk for cardiovascular disease.

b. Population: Military men and women
c. Setting: Outpatient primary care clinic of a 140-bed military hospital.

5. The study was feasible because of the availability of a large number of subjects through the outpatient clinic. In addition, the military hospital provided the equipment and facility needed to conduct the study and supported the lipid lab work that was done before and after the educational program. The researchers demonstrated the educational preparation and clinical expertise to conduct this study. The study was conducted ethically with the protection of subjects' rights.

Making Connections

Objectives, Questions, and Hypotheses

1. b, c, d, g
2. a, c, e, g
3. b, c, e, f
4. a, d, g, h
5. b, d, g, h
6. b, c, d, g
7. a, c, e, g
8. b, c, e, f
9. a, c, e, g
10. b, d, g, h
11. Low-back massage is no more effective in decreasing perceptions of low-back pain than no massage in patients with chronic low-back pain.
12. Increased age, decreased family support, and decreased health status are related to decreased self-care abilities of nursing home residents.
13. Nurses' perceived work stress, internal locus of control, and social support are not related to their psychological symptoms.

Exercises in Critique

Carey et al. Study

This study had no objectives, questions, or hypotheses. The purpose for this study had two parts that directed the conduct of this study.

Lewis et al. Study

1. Research questions: "1. Does the change in SvO_2 after a 1-minute backrub in critically ill patients given the backrub immediately after turning differ from the change in SvO_2 in patients given the backrub 5 minutes after turning? 2. What is the effect of right and left lateral positions on SvO_2 in critically ill patients?" (p. 218)

2. The questions are clearly stated, reflective of the purpose, and provide direction for the conduct of the study. Since this is a quasi-experimental study, the authors might have provided clearer direction for their study with the statement of hypotheses versus research questions.

Bruce and Grove Study

1. Research question: "What is the difference in the mean total serum cholesterol, LDL cholesterol, and HDL cholesterol and cardiovascular risk levels of military members before and after participation in the C.A.R.E. program?" (Bruce & Grove, 1994, p. 233).
2. This question is clearly stated, includes the appropriate study variables, and directs the remaining steps of the research process.

Making Connections

Understanding Study Variables

1. a
2. b
3. c
4. a
5. b
6. b
7. c
8. c
9. a
10. b
11. a
12. a

Exercises in Critique

Carey et al. Study

1. Independent variable: Group assignment was identified as the independent variable (mothers with healthy children and mothers with children with CHD).
   Dependent variables: Child-rearing practices, parenting stress, parental expectations, and behavioral and emotional development were identified as dependent variables. However, since this was an exploratory and descriptive study, these might be best identified as research variables.
2. Research variable: Parenting stress
   Conceptual definition: Type of parental response to a young child that would vary based on whether the child was healthy or had a chronic illness. No clear conceptual definition is provided in the article. The definition was abstracted from the framework on pp. 199-200 of the study.
   Operational definition: "The Parenting Stress Index-Short Form (PSI) is a 36-item, self-report measure of the amount of stress experienced by parents of young children (Abidin, 1995). The PSI measures parenting stress on three subscales:

(1) parent distress . . .; (2) parent-child dysfunctional interaction . . .; and (3) difficult child . . ." (pp. 201-202).
Research variable: Behavioral and emotional development
Conceptual definition: "How parents respond [overprotective or authoritative parenting style] over time can influence the children's short- and long-term developmental outcomes" (p. 198).
Operational definition: "The Eyberg Child Behavior Inventory (ECBI; Eyberg & Ross, 1978) is a 36-item inventory that measures behavior problems common to children 2 to 16 years old . . . The Behavioral Screening Questionnaire (BSQ; Richman & Graham, 1971) is a screening tool used to identify behavioral and emotional problems in preschool children" (p. 202).

3. The conceptual definition of parenting stress must be abstracted from the framework for the study. The concept of parental responses can be linked to the variable parenting stress. The operational definition of parenting stress is clearly expressed in the article and provides quality measurement of the variable. The conceptual and operational definitions for behavioral and emotional development are clearly expressed in the article. The conceptual definition provides a basis for the operational definition, and the operational definition clearly identifies the two scales that will be used to measure this variable.

Lewis et al. Study

1. Independent variables: Body position (right or left lateral) and timing of backrub (immediate or delayed)
   Dependent variable: Mixed venous oxygen saturation (SvO_2)
2. Independent variable: Body position
   Conceptual definition: "Nursing intervention to promote patients' comfort, mobilizing pulmonary secretions, and improving tissue perfusion through pressure reduction . . . Routine nursing care such as turning the patient, suctioning, weighing, bed baths, and backrubs may cause increased oxygen consumption" (p. 218).
   Operational definition: Intervention where the "patient was turned to the left or right lateral position. A single data collector turned the patient and placed two folded standard pillows, one pillow behind the patient's back and one between the patient's knees" (p. 222).
3. Conceptual definition is abstracted from the problem and the study framework. The operational definition is clearly expressed and controlled in implementation by one data collector who did all the patient body positioning.

Bruce and Grove Study

1. Independent variable: C.A.R.E. program
   Dependent variables: Total cholesterol, HDL, LDL, and cardiovascular risk level
2. C.A.R.E. program
   Conceptual definition: Health screening and educational program designed to effect positive health outcomes (reduction in CAD risk) in people.
   Operational definition: The C.A.R.E. program was implemented according to the guidelines in Figure 1 of the article (Bruce & Grove, 1994, p. 234).
3. The conceptual and operational definitions of the C.A.R.E. program are clearly presented in the article. All the dependent variables are clearly operationally defined but the conceptual definitions might have been clearer.

CHAPTER 4—LITERATURE REVIEW

Relevant Terms

1. m
2. j
3. p
4. q
5. e
6. k
7. n
8. d
9. i
10. c
11. l
12. o
13. r
14. h
15. g
16. a
17. b
18. f

Key Ideas

1. theoretical and empirical sources
2. compare and combine findings from the study with the literature to determine current knowledge of a phenomenon
3. ethnographic and quantitative research (descriptive, correlational, quasi-experimental, and experimental studies)
4. historical research
5. landmark
6. known and not known
7. published 5 to 10 years before publication of the report
8. secondary source
9. electronic databases
10. Internet

11. a. selecting databases to search
    b. selecting keywords
    c. locating relevant literature
    d. storing references using reference management software
12. Cumulative Index to Nursing & Allied Health Literature (CINAHL)
13. thesaurus
14. store information retrieved from computer reference databases
15. *Annual Review of Nursing Research*
16. synthesis
17. introduction, empirical literature, and summary
18. Key terms to direct the literature review include core rewarming, cardiac surgery rewarming, radiant heat rewarming, forced air rewarming, rewarming after surgery, peripheral hypothermia, vasoconstriction, and postoperative period.
19. Key terms to direct the literature review include urinary incontinence, daytime incontinence, nighttime incontinence, urinary incontinence management, prompted voiding, and nursing home residents.
20. a. the name of the database used
    b. the date the search is performed
    c. the exact search strategy that is used
    d. the number of articles that are found
    e. the percentage of relevant articles that are found

Making Connections

Theoretical and Empirical Sources

1. T
2. E
3. E
4. T
5. T
6. E
7. E
8. E
9. T
10. T
11. E

Primary and Secondary Sources

1. S
2. P
3. P
4. S
5. S
6. P
7. P
8. S
9. P
10. P

Exercises in Critique

1. a. name of the journal
   b. year the study was published
   c. volume number of the journal
   d. pages of the article
   e. issue number of the journal
   f. Bruce and Grove
   g. The effect of a coronary artery risk evaluation program on serum lipid values and cardiovascular risk levels.
2. Carey, L. K., Nicholson, B. C., & Fox, R. A. (2002). Maternal factors related to parenting young children with congenital heart disease. *Journal of Pediatric Nursing, 17*(3), 174-183.
3. a. title and pages of the article
   b. volume number of the journal and pages of the article
   c. year the article was published and volume and issue numbers of the journal
4. a. Review of the Literature
   b. Literature Review
   c. Background
5. Yes, relevant studies are identified and described. By examining the literature review section and the references of the Carey et al. (2002) study, it appears that they identified and described at least six relevant studies in their literature review: DeMaso, Beardslee, Silbert, & Fyler, 1991; Goldberg, Simmons, Newman, Campbell, & Fowler, 1991; Krulik, 1980; Lobo, 1992; Marino & Lipshitz, 1991; Svavarstottir & McCummin, 1996.
6. Carey et al. (2002) state the proposition that the family context is an important contributing factor in the socialization of children. Two theoretical sources cited to support this proposition are Maccoby, 1992 and Maccoby & Martin, 1983.
7. primary source
8. Austin, J. K. (1991). Family adaptation to a child's chronic illness. *Annual Review of Nursing Research, 9*, 103-120.
9. The Carey et al. study was published in 2002. There is no indication in the article of when the study was originally submitted or accepted for publication. At the end of the paper, an acknowledgment indicates that "This research served as the basis for the first author's doctoral dissertation and was supported in part by a grant from the Children's Hospital Foundation, Milwaukee, WI" (p. 213). However, Carey's dissertation is not cited in the references, and thus, there is no indication of when the dissertation was completed. A CINAHL search revealed that Carey's dissertation was completed in 1999 at Marquette University. The average span of time between submission of an article and publication is 2 years. Therefore, an estimate of submission date might be 2000. The paper appears to have been completed within a year of finishing the dissertation. The references range

from 1971 through 2000. Therefore, it is apparent that the authors continued to search for new literature until the paper was submitted for publication. The sources cited seem relevant to the topic, and 28 of the 41 sources or 68% were published in the 10 years prior to publication. Thus, one can be justified in judging that the references are current.

10. A search of CINAHL in August, 2002 using the keyword (1) HEART DEFECTS, CONGENITAL yielded 480 hits. A second search of keywords (2) ALTERED PARENTING or CARETAKING/PARENTING or PARENTING ALTERATION or PARENTING: SOCIAL SAFETY or RISK OF ALTERED PARENTING yielded 1064 hits. Combining the two sets of keywords yielded 4 hits. A third search using keywords (3) MATERNAL ATTITUDES or MATERNAL ROLE or MATERNAL BEHAVIOR or MATERNAL-CHILD CARE yielded 2201 hits. Combining searches 1 and 3 yielded 3 hits. This information suggests that previous studies examining parenting of young children with congenital heart disease are limited and that the article by Carey et al. (2002) probably does represent the current knowledge base in this field of research.
11. Yes, relevant studies are identified and described. By examining the Lewis et al. (1997) Literature Review Section and References, there appear to be at least 10 studies cited. Some of the research sources include Shively, 1988; Tidwell, Ryan, Osguthorpe, Paull, & Smith, 1990; Winslow, Clark, White, & Tyler, 1990; Copel & Stolarik, 1991; Atkins, Hapshe, & Riegel, 1994; Tyler, Winslow, Clark, & White, 1990.
12. Lewis et al. (1997) indicated the framework for their study was based on the physiological principles underlying SvO_2. They cited three theoretical sources that were physiologically focused in their Framework Section: Ahrens & Rutherford, 1993; Cernaianu & Nelson, 1993; White, Winslow, Clark, & Tyler, 1990
13. secondary source, primary source
14. The Lewis et al. (1997) study has current sources. The references ranged from 1982 through 1994 and the article was published in early 1997. There is no indication when the article was submitted or accepted for publication, which might account for the last reference being published in 1994. Nine of the 15 sources, or 60%, were published in the 1990s, and four of these were published in 1993-1994.
15. Lewis et al. (1997) provide detailed coverage of relevant studies (pp. 219-221) and also a clear summary of what is known. "In summary, nursing interventions cause a significant decrease in SvO_2 immediately after the intervention is started. SvO_2 values usually return to baseline within 3 to 9 minutes, depending on the intervention" (p. 221). However, their review of literature would have been stronger if they had indicated what is not known and how their study will contribute to the development of nursing knowledge in the area studied.
16. By examining the background section and the references of the Bruce and Grove article, you will note that they identified and described 15 studies. Some of those studies were Blair, Bryant, & Bocuzzi (1988); Blankenhorn, Nessim, Johnson,

San Marco, Azen, & Cashen-Hemphill (1987); Bruno, Arnold, Winick, & Wynder (1983); Freidewald, Levy, & Fredrickson (1972); Lipid Research Clinics Program (1984).

17. Bruce and Grove (1994) cited physiological, pathological, and health education theoretical sources to support their study. Some of the theoretical sources include American Heart Association (1988); Green, Kreuter, Deeds, & Partiridge (1980); Kwiterovick (1989). Some of the theoretical content and sources were deleted at the request of the journal editor to shorten the article and increase the appeal to the journal audience.
18. secondary source, primary source
19. The references range from 1947 through 1990. The article was published in 1994, so the authors' sources are at least 4 years old. However, this article was submitted in 1992, accepted for publication in 1993, and published in 1994. The delay between submitting the article and publication can make some of the references less current. Over 50% of the sources were from the late 1980s.
20. Bruce and Grove clearly summarize what is known and not known about the effects of educational programs on adults' serum lipid values and cardiovascular risk levels. The study by Blair, Bryant, and Bocuzzi (1988) highlights the effectiveness of nursing intervention in individuals with hyperlipidemia. The authors indicate how their study will add to the current knowledge base in this area of study.

CHAPTER 5—UNDERSTANDING THEORY AND RESEARCH FRAMEWORKS

Relevant Terms

Check the glossary in the back of your text for definitions.

Key Ideas

1. to organize what we know about a phenomenon
2. determining the truth of each relational statement in the theory
3. Conceptual models
4. theory
5. disconnected
6. the framework
7. concepts
8. constructs
9. variable
10. propositions
11. hypotheses

12. explain which concepts contribute to or partially cause an outcome
13. all of the major concepts in a theory or framework linked together by arrows expressing the proposed linkages between the concepts
14. research tradition

Making Connections

1. e
2. b
3. a
4. h
5. c
6. d
7. i
8. g
9. f

Exercises in Critique

1. Concepts
   - SvO_2
   - oxygen supply
   - tissue oxygen demands
   - SaO_2
   - hemoglobin level
   - cardiac output
   - tissue oxygen consumption
   - routine nursing care
   - patient conditions
2. Conceptual definitions
   - SvO_2—mixed venous oxygen saturation
   - oxygen supply—not defined
   - tissue oxygen demand—not defined
   - SaO_2—arterial oxygen saturation
   - hemoglobin level—not defined
   - cardiac output—not defined
   - tissue oxygen consumption—not defined
   - routine nursing care—not defined
   - patient conditions—not defined

3. Table of Concepts, Related Variables, and Measurement Methods

Concept	Variable	Measurement
SvO_2	SvO_2	fiber-optic thermodilution pulmonary artery catheter measures
oxygen supply		
tissue oxygen demand		
SaO_2		
hemoglobin level		
cardiac output		
tissue oxygen consumption		
routine nursing care	position of patient	turning patient to right or left
	immediacy of backrub	immediate or delayed backrub
patient conditions		

4. Measurement methods are consistent with concepts. However, conceptual definitions are not provided and cannot be compared.
5. An uncompensated reduction in SaO_2, hemoglobin level, or cardiac output or increases in tissue oxygen consumption will result in a decreased SvO_2.

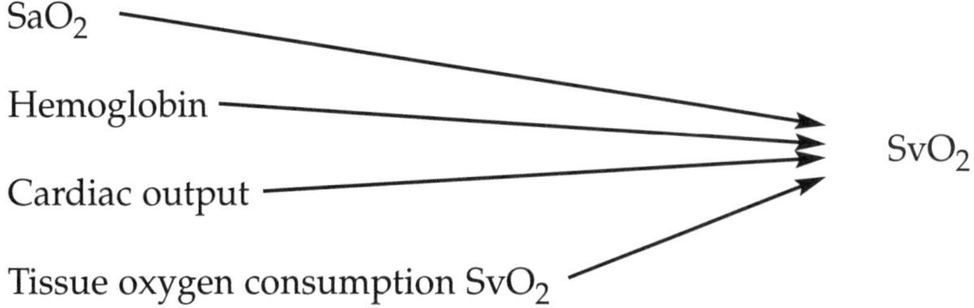

The SaO_2 influences the SvO_2.

SaO_2 ——→ SvO_2

Pathological pulmonary conditions that impair oxygen transfer at the alveolar-capillary membrane will result in less oxygen available for transport through the circulation.

Patient condition ——→ oxygen supply

A deficit in hemoglobin reduces the oxygen-binding capacity of the blood and affects oxygen supply to the tissues.

Hemoglobin ——→ oxygen supply

Cardiac output is the means for transporting oxyhemoglobin through the system.

Cardiac output ——→ oxygen supply

Tissue extraction of oxygen is increased in conditions such as fever, seizures, and shivering.

Patient condition ——→ tissue oxygen consumption

Routine nursing care such as turning the patient, suctioning, weighing, bed baths, and backrubs may cause increased oxygen consumption.

Routine nursing care ——→ tissue oxygen consumption

6. Proposition: Routine nursing care such as turning the patient, suctioning, weighing, bed baths, and backrubs may cause increased oxygen consumption.
   Research question: Does the change in SvO_2 after a 1-minute backrub in critically ill patients given the backrub immediately after turning differ from the change in SvO_2 in patients given the backrub 5 minutes after turning?
   Research question: What is the effect of right and left lateral positions in SvO_2 in critically ill patients?
7. The proposition is tested by the study design by testing differences in the effect of providing backrubs immediately after turning and 5 minutes after turning and differences in the effect of turning the patient to the right and to the left.

8. The framework is not expressed as a conceptual map. A possible map of the framework is shown below:

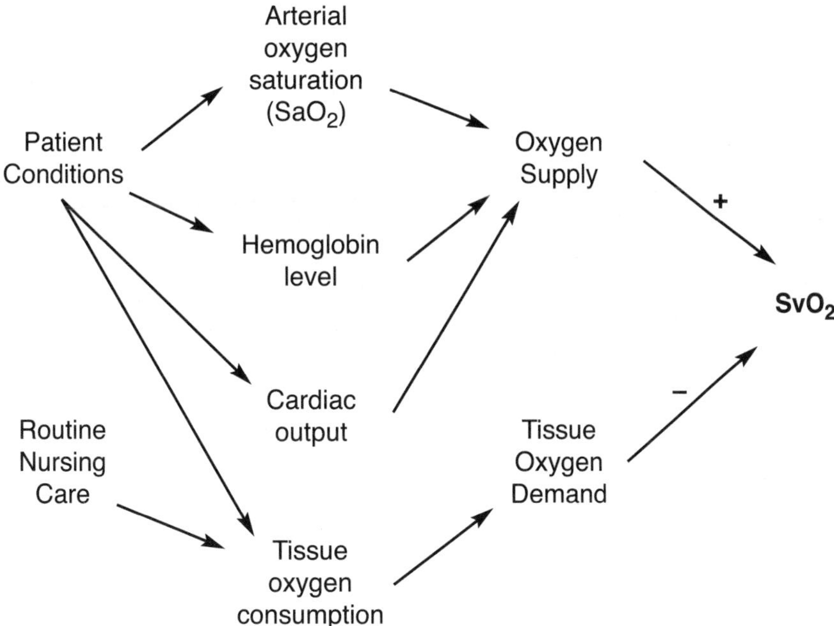

9. References from the literature
   Effects of nursing care on oxygen consumption
      Shively (1988)
      Tidwell, Ryan, Psguthorpe, Paull, & Smith (1990)
      Winslow, Clark, & White (1990)
      Copel & Stolarik (1991)
      Atkins, Hapshe, & Riegel (1994)
      Tyler, Winslow, Clark, & White (1990)
   No other relationships validated from the literature
10. Paragraphs will vary but should include the following points:
    The framework expresses the causal linkages associated with SvO_2. Conceptual definitions are not provided. This commonly occurs with physiologic concepts because the concepts are assumed by the author to have a common meaning that will be known by the readers. Relationships between concepts are not presented in theoretical form and are somewhat difficult to sort out from the discussion provided. No conceptual map is provided.

CHAPTER 6—EXAMINING ETHICS IN NURSING RESEARCH

Relevant Terms

1. f
2. a
3. g
4. i
5. h
6. d
7. j
8. b
9. l
10. e
11. c
12. k

Key Ideas

1. a. Disclosure of essential study information to the subject
   b. Comprehension of this information by the subject
   c. Competency of the subject to give consent
   d. Voluntary consent by the subject to participate in the study
2. You might have identified any of the following:
   a. Introduction of the research activities
   b. Statement of the research purpose
   c. Explanation of study procedures
   d. Description of risks and discomforts
   e. Description of benefits
   f. Disclosure of alternatives
   g. Assurance of anonymity and confidentiality
   h. Offer to answer questions
   i. Option to withdraw
3. Voluntary
4. incompetent
5. Institutional Review Board (IRB)
6. a. Exempt from review
   b. Expedited review
   c. Complete or full review
7. To determine the benefit-risk ratio, you need to assess the benefits and risks of the sampling method, consent process, procedures, and outcomes of the study. Informed consent must be obtained from the subjects, and selection and treatment of the subjects during the study must be fair. The type of knowledge generated from the study also needs to be examined to determine how this knowledge will impact the subject and influence nursing practice. The risks need to be reduced, if possible, and should not cause serious harm to the subjects; the benefits need to be maximized. Then the risks and the benefits are examined; the benefits need to adequately outweigh the risks for the study to be considered ethical to conduct.

8. Exempt from review or expedited review
9. Complete review
10. Possible answers: fabrication, falsification, or forging of data; manipulation of the design or methods; selective retaining or manipulating data; or plagiarism.
11. Office of Scientific Integrity Review (OSIR) and Office of Scientific Integrity (OSI)
12. Yes. This is an area of concern in nursing, and articles have been published outlining the concerns and actions to be taken to control scientific misconduct. None of the major misconduct problems mentioned in the text has been in nursing.
13. Yes. An increasing number of animals are being used by nurse scientists to generate basic research knowledge for the profession.
14. American Association for Accreditation of Laboratory Animal Care (AAALAC)
15. Best answer is yes. Rationale might focus on the importance of animal studies to generate basic knowledge to provide a basis for conducting applied studies on humans. Agencies exist to protect the animals and ensure humane treatment during research.
    If you answered no, your rationale might focus on the inhuman aspects of using animals in studies.

Making Connections

Historical Events, Ethical Codes, and Regulations

1. b
2. c
3. d
4. b
5. c
6. a
7. d
8. b
9. a
10. c

Puzzle

Crossword Puzzle

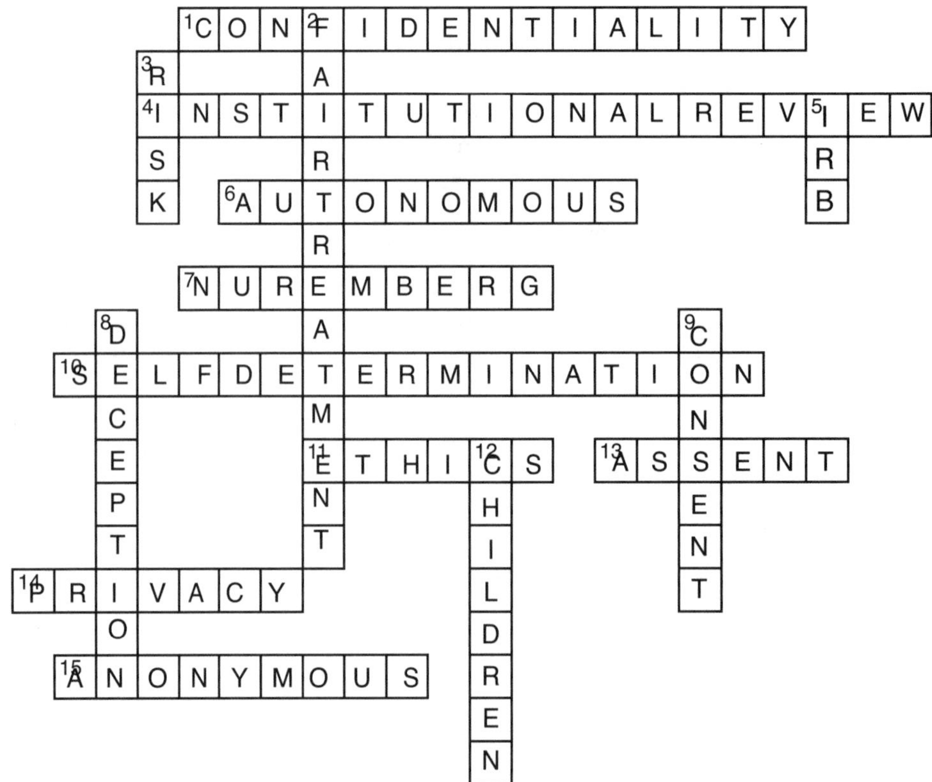

Exercises in Critique

1. Carey et al. (2002) study was ethical as indicated by the following excerpt from the article: "Subjects who met the inclusion criteria were visited in their homes by the first author who reviewed the study procedures and obtained written informed consent. The home visits averaged about 1.5 hours in length. Mothers received $50 for participating and their children were given a toy or book" (p. 201). There is no indication that the study was reviewed by an Institutional Review Board (IRB) for the University, but I am sure this occurred since this study was the dissertation for Carey. This study appears to be ethical when examining the benefit-risk ratio, but the authors might have provided more information about the approval process for conducting this study.

2. Lewis et al. (1997) identified the following ethical process for obtaining subject's consent to participate in their study: "The study was approved by the institutional review board, and all subjects signed an informed consent document" (p. 221). The authors discussed their approval by an Institutional Review Board. This study appears to be ethical, since the risks are minimal and the benefits are strong and the authors indicated signed consent forms were obtained from the subjects.
3. Bruce & Grove (1994) indicated that the Strategic Air Command Surgeon General mandated the educational program (institutional review) be provided to the military members and dependents and participation in the study was voluntary (p. 233). The study was ethical because the researchers obtained institutional approval and signed consent from the subjects, who voluntarily participated in the study. In addition, the risks were minimal and the benefits were strong in this study.

CHAPTER 7—CLARIFYING RESEARCH DESIGNS

Relevant Terms

Check the glossary in the back of your text for definitions.

Key Ideas

1. effects
2. cause; effect; cause
3. biases
4. control
5. treatment
6. threats to validity
7. cause and effect
8. comparisons
9. comparisons

Making Connections

Matching Definitions

1. g
2. h
3. i
4. a
5. f
6. c
7. d
8. b
9. e

Matching Designs

1. a
2. c
3. f
4. g
5. b
6. j
7. e
8. i
9. h
10. d

Mapping the Design

1. **Home Care for Terminal Cancer Patients**

	1 Week Before	Hospital Discharge	1 Week After	4 Weeks After	Death	3 Months After
Exp Grp		Experimental Intervention				
Obs	O_1		O_2	O_3		O_4
Comp Grp		Standard Care				
Obs	O_1		O_2	O_3		O_4

2. **Communication with Families in an ICU**

Admission	24 Hours Later		Discharge from ICU or 2 Weeks After Admission
Exp Grp	O_1	Experimental Intervention	O_2
Comp Grp	O_1	Standard Care	O_2

Exercises in Critique

1. Design
   a. Carey et al. study—descriptive comparative.
   b. Lewis et al. study—according to the criteria in this text, this is a quasi-experimental study; the author's refer to it as experimental.
   c. Bruce & Grove study—descriptive comparative.
2. Sources of bias
   a. Carey et al. study
      1. Mothers of children with congenital heart disease were recruited at a large pediatric cardiology clinic at a children's hospital. Mothers of healthy children were recruited from pediatric medical practices and school settings and matched with the first group based on the child's age and gender, and mother's marital and socioeconomic status. Subjects who volunteered may have been different from those who did not volunteer. For example, those who volunteered may have been more invested in their children than those who did not express interest in the study. The authors do not address whether the sample is representative of the target population, which seems to be the dyad of mother and preschool child with a chronic disease.
      2. Out of 36 mothers with a child with congenital heart disease who were invited to participate in the study, 6 declined for personal reasons, a 17% refusal rate. The authors do not report the refusal rate among the mothers with healthy children. As the refusal rate increases, the risk of biases in the sample increase.
      3. The sample size is small, increasing the risks of nonrepresentativeness.
      4. Mothers of children with congenital heart disease were less likely to be working out of the home than mothers of healthy children, which could effect the mother-child relationship being studied.

b. Lewis et al. study
   1. Sample was not randomly selected. Subjects volunteering may have been different from those who did not volunteer.
   2. The sample included only males, a consequence of conducting the study at a Veteran's Administration hospital.
   3. Other than gender, the author does not address whether the sample is representative of people being cared for in a surgical ICU.

c. Bruce & Grove study
   1. Sample was not randomly selected. Subjects volunteering may have been different from those who did not volunteer.
   2. Ethnicity of the sample is not reported, thus the possibility of bias cannot be judged. The effectiveness of risk-reduction strategies may differ in some ethnic groups due to genetic variation.
   3. Military personnel may differ from the general population in the likelihood that they will follow a risk-reduction program.

3. Methods of control
   a. Carey et al. study—You could have listed any three of the following:
      1. Controlling equivalence—Matching of subjects in the comparison groups is a powerful way to reduce bias.
      2. Controlling equivalence—The use of a severity of congenital heart disease score as a sampling criteria increased the comparability of the chronically ill children.
      3. Controlling measurement—Instruments with documented validity and reliability were used for measurement.
      4. Controlling measurement—A single data collector performed all of the observations and measurements.
      5. Detailed descriptive data were gathered on subjects to identify potential extraneous variables.
   b. Lewis et al. study—You could have listed any three of the following:
      1. Controlling measurement—Valid and reliable instruments were used. Physiologic measures were carefully controlled for consistency.
      2. Controlling extraneous variables—Potential subjects were excluded if they were less than 18 years of age; had sepsis; had had pneumonectory, lobectomy, or organ transplantation; had mechanical assist devices in place, or were using neuromuscular blocking agents.
      3. A nested design was used to examine interactions of turning and backrub.
      4. Intervention—The procedures for turning and backrub were carefully defined.
      5. A single data collector provided the intervention and collected the data for a patient.

c. Bruce & Grove study—You could have listed any three of the following:
   1. Controlling the environment—Subjects received a carefully designed treatment at one military base.
   2. Controlling equivalence—Subjects were limited to those with serum cholesterol levels between 200 mg/dl and 300 mg/dl.
   3. Controlling treatment—A defined protocol was used as the treatment.
   4. Controlling measurement—A standardized protocol for lipid data collection was followed by each subject.
   5. Subjects were excluded if they were diabetic or were being pharmacologically treated for hyperlipidemia.

4. Comparisons
   a. Carey et al. study
      1. Comparison of maternal expectations
      2. Comparison of maternal discipline
      3. Comparison of maternal nurturing
      4. Comparison of maternal distress
      5. Comparison of maternal-child dysfunction
      6. Comparison of child behavior intensity
      7. Comparison of child behavior frequency
      8. Comparison of child problem behaviors
      9. Comparison of child prosocial behaviors
      10. Comparison of parent positives
      11. Comparison of parent negatives
      12. Comparison of child negatives
      13. Comparison of total commands by mother
      14. Comparison of total compliant behaviors by child
      15. Comparison of total noncompliant behaviors by child
   b. Lewis et al. study
      1. Comparisons across timed measurements for each subject
      2. Comparisons of baseline values between the two groups
      3. Comparisons of left turns and right turns between the two groups and for the total sample.
      4. Comparisons of timing of backrub between the two groups and for the total sample.
      5. Comparisons of the effect of turns and the effect of backrub for the total sample.
   c. Bruce & Grove study
      1. Risk levels of subjects before and after treatment using a standard protocol
      2. Comparison of cardiovascular risk and total cholesterol level
      3. Comparison of cardiovascular risk and LDL cholesterol
      4. Comparison of cardiovascular risk and HDL cholesterol

5. Generalizations
   a. Carey et al. study
      1. Generalized to normal developmental expectations.
         Children with congenital heart disease could not be distinguished from healthy children by their behavior.
   b. Lewis et al. study
      1. Male patients being cared for in a surgical ICU who are similar to subjects in the study.
      2. ICU patients receiving a backrub using the same procedure as that used in the study.
      3. ICU patients being turned using the same procedure as that used in the study.
      4. ICU patients with SvO_2 values similar to those of subjects in the study.
      5. ICU patients with hemoglobin levels similar to those of subjects in the study.
      6. ICU patients with hemodynamically stable conditions.
   c. Bruce & Grove's study
      1. Cardiovascular high-risk patients
6. Threats to external validity
   a. Carey et al. study
      1. Convenience sample
      2. Small sample size
   b. Lewis et al. study
      1. Interaction of selection and treatment—Only patients who were hemodynamically stable were included in the study. The treatment may not have the same effect on patients who are unstable.
   c. Bruce & Grove study
      1. Interaction of selection and treatment—Because compliance of military personnel to treatment may be higher than that of general public.
7. Strengths of the design
   a. Carey et al. study
      1. Matching of subjects
      2. Excellence of measurement methods
      3. Design guided by theoretical testing
   b. Lewis et al. study
      1. Random assignment of subjects to groups
      2. Repeated measures
      3. Controlled treatment
   c. Bruce & Grove study
      1. Carefully designed protocol
      2. Large sample size
      3. Control of measurement

CHAPTER 8—POPULATIONS AND SAMPLES

Relevant Terms

1. j
2. a
3. n
4. g
5. k
6. f
7. m
8. i
9. l
10. b
11. d
12. e
13. h
14. c

Key Ideas

1. elements
2. target population
3. sample, accessible population, and target population
4. You might identify any two of the following:
   a. Compare the demographic characteristics of the sample with those of the target population.
   b. Compare mean sample values of study variables with the values of the target population determined from previous research.
   c. Determine sample mortality.
   d. Evaluate the possibilities of systematic bias in the sample in terms of the setting, characteristics of the sample, and ranges of values on measured variables.
5. the expected difference in values that occurs when different subjects from the same sample are examined
6. sampling frame
7. strategies used to obtain a sample for a study
8. You might choose any of the following.
   a. Did the researcher successfully implement the sampling plan?
   b. Was the sampling plan effective in achieving representativeness?
   c. Were the subjects selected from a sampling frame?
   d. Were the subjects randomly selected?
   e. If control and treatment groups were used, how were these groups selected?
9. homogeneous
10. heterogenous
11. sample criteria
12. sample characteristics
13. sample mortality
14. random

15. nonrandom
16. a. simple random sampling
    b. stratified random sampling
    c. cluster sampling
    d. systematic sampling
17. probability
18. a. convenience sampling
    b. quota sampling
    c. purposive sampling
    d. network sampling
19. nonprobability
20. accidental sampling
21. judgmental sampling
22. power analysis
23. differences or relationships
24. 0.8
25. power analysis
26. null hypothesis
27. a. effect size of a study
    b. type of study
    c. number of variables
    d. measurement sensitivity
    e. data analysis techniques

Making Connections

1. f
2. b
3. c
4. a
5. b
6. g
7. h
8. b
9. e
10. d
11. f
12. c
13. d
14. b
15. f

Puzzle

Crossword Puzzle

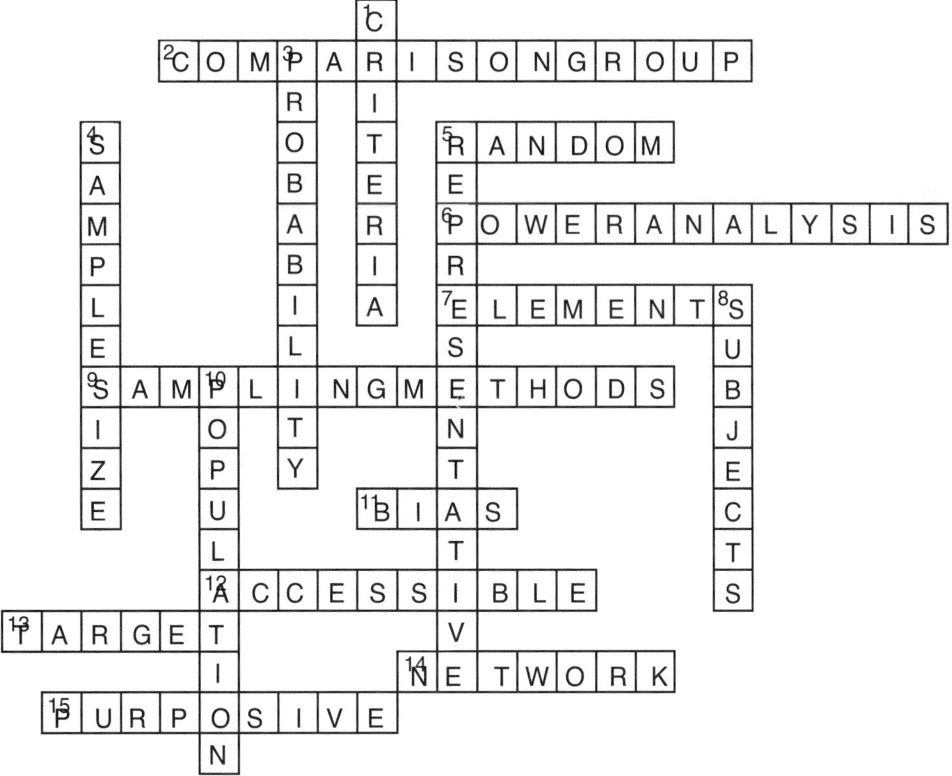

Exercises in Critique

Bruce and Grove Study

1. Sample criteria: "(a) greater than 16 years; (b) military members (active duty, retired, or dependent); (c) not under pharmacological treatment for hyperlipidemia; (d) English-speaking; (e) triglycerides under 400 mg/dl . . .; (f) nondiabetic; and (g) no current referrals to other health providers" (Bruce & Grove, 1994, p. 235).
2. Sample characteristics: "The sample consisted of 92 men and 103 women and included 36 married couples. The subjects ranged from 20 to 80 years of age, with a mean age of 53.33 years (+ 13 SD). Information about the subjects' body mass index (BMI), systolic blood pressure (SBP), diastolic blood pressure (DBP), heart rate, and glucose are provided in Table 1. Means for these variables were within normal limits" (Bruce & Grove, 1994, p. 235).

3. Sample size: 195. "A power analysis was performed to confirm the adequacy of the sample size" (Bruce & Grove, 1994, p. 235). However, the specifics of this analysis were deleted from the article at the request of the journal editor.
4. The sample size was adequate to examine four variables in this quasi-experimental study. Power analysis indicated that the sample size was adequate to detect differences. Very sensitive measurements were obtained of the total cholesterol, HDL, and LDL.
5. No sample mortality. A total of 483 subjects were screened, but only 195 became subjects and completed the study.
6. nonprobability
7. convenience sampling
8. Since the sample is nonrandom, this has a potential to decrease its representativeness of the population. However, actively recruiting subjects and including all subjects that met the sample criteria increases the representativeness of this sample. The large sample size increases the representativeness of the sample.
9. Since the sample is nonrandom, the findings should be generalized to the accessible population and not the target population. However, since these findings are extremely consistent with the extensive number of studies in this area, this increases the generalizability of the findings.

Carey et al. Study

1. Sample criteria: "mothers of young children [2 to 5 years of age] with moderated to severe CHD [coronary heart disease]" and "mothers of healthy children (absence of chronic illnesses, significant health conditions, or birth anomalies)" (p. 200).
2. Sample characteristics: "For the CHD group, children's mean age was 3.44 years (SD = 0.93), mothers' mean age was 33.5 years (SD = 4.45), and the family included an average of 2.03 children (range = 1-5). For the healthy group, children's mean age was 3.43 years (SD = 0.94), mothers' mean age was 32.13 years (SD = 4.16), and the family included an average of 2.20 children (range = 1-4). Additional demographic data for the study groups are shown in Table 1" (p. 202). (See article in Appendix B for Table 1.)
3. Sample size: 60 subjects
4. The sample size does not appear to be adequate. No power analysis was done to determine the sample size needed for the study. Many of the findings were nonsignificant and might be due to the small sample size resulting in Type II errors (saying something is nonsignificant when it is significant). This is a descriptive study that involves measurement of several variables and needed a larger sample size to detect differences between the groups. A larger sample would have allowed testing for a smaller effect size.

5. 60 subjects (30 in each group) comprised the final sample. No sample mortality was identified. All analyses were conducted on the data from 60 subjects.
6. nonprobability sample
7. convenience sampling
8. Since the sample was not random, this decreases its probability of being representative of the population. "The sample of 30 mothers of healthy children was matched with the CHD sample based on the children's age and gender and the maternal marital and socioeconomic status" (p. 202). The matching decreases influence of these matched variables on the study findings and decreases sampling error. The subjects were of varied educational levels, family income, social support, and professional and nonprofessional work status, making the sample more reflective of the population. However, the sample was predominately Caucasian, which decreases the representativeness of the sample. Based on the sample size, sampling method, and some of the sample characteristics, this sample is not representative of the population, and the authors need to limit their generalization of their findings.
9. Since this is a nonrandom sample that does not appear to be representative, the findings should be generalized to the accessible population and not the target population.

Lewis et al. Study

1. Sample criteria: "Subjects who had a fiber-optic pulmonary artery catheter in place, a baseline SvO_2 of 50% or higher, and an indwelling arterial catheter with normal waveform were eligible for inclusion in the study. Exclusion criteria included age less than 18 years, sepsis, pneumonectomy or lobectomy, mechanical assist devices in place, organ transplantation, and use of neuromuscular blocking agents. No subjects were exclude because of advanced age" (p. 221).
2. Sample characteristics: "The mean age of the subjects was 60.9 years (standard deviation [SD] = 8.6; range = 40-79 years). Forty-nine subjects had had aortocoronary bypass surgery; 6, resection of an aortic aneurysm; 1, atrial septal repair; and 1, an esophogastrectomy. All subjects were in the surgical ICU at the time of the intervention. Forty-nine subjects were receiving oxygen by either face mask (n = 22) or nasal cannula (n = 27). Four subjects were receiving mechanical ventilation; 3 of these were receiving 5 cm of positive end-expiratory pressure. The remaining 4 subjects had no supplemental oxygen therapy. Mean SaO_2, hemoglobin, cardiac output, and cardiac index are given in Table 1" (p. 223). (Table 1 is provided in the article in Appendix B).
3. Sample size: 57 subjects. "Power analysis for repeated measures indicates that 23 subjects are needed to detect a medium effect at the 0.05 level of significance with a power of 0.80 and an estimated mean correlation among the repeated measures of 0.50 when only seven repeated measures are collected. This study had two

grouping variables: position and immediacy of backrub. A minimum of 23 subjects was recruited into each group. This sample size provided more than adequate power, because 15 repeated measures were recorded for each subject" (p. 221).
4. The study hypotheses were supported, and the sample size was adequate.
5. No sample mortality is reported.
6. nonprobability
7. convenience sampling
8. Since the sample was not random, this decreases its representativeness of the population studied. Women were not included in the sample, which decreases the sample's representativeness. The authors point out that only hemodynamically stable patients were included in the sample.
9. Since the sample is nonrandom, the findings need to be generalized to the accessible population. However, since these findings were consistent with the findings of other studies, this increases the generalizability of the findings. The findings cannot be generalized to women or to patients who are hemodynamically unstable.

CHAPTER 9—MEASUREMENT AND DATA COLLECTION IN RESEARCH

Relevant Terms

Define terms using the glossary in your textbook.

Key Ideas

1. trustworthy
2. true
3. error
4. direct
5. indirect
6. 0.80

Random Error

1. Variations in administration of the measurement procedure
2. Subjects completing a paper and pencil scale accidentally marking the wrong column
3. Punching the wrong key while entering data into the computer

Systematic Error

1. A weight scale that weighs higher than it should
2. A thermometer that is not calibrated
3. Failure to count two exam questions in calculating exam grades

Data Collection Tasks

1. Selecting subjects
2. Collecting data in a consistent way
3. Maintaining research controls indicated by the study design
4. Protecting the study integrity (or validity)
5. Solving problems that threaten to disrupt the study

Making Connections

Measurement Error

1. b
2. b
3. a
4. b
5. a

Level of Measurement

1. c
2. a
3. b
4. c
5. a
6. b
7. c

Type of Reliability or Validity

1. g
2. d
3. k
4. m
5. e
6. a
7. h
8. c
9. i
10. j
11. f
12. l
13. b

Exercises in Critique

Matching Variables

Carey et al. study

Variable	Method of Measurement	Directness
Expectations	Parent Behavior Checklist	I
Discipline	Parent Behavior Checklist	I
Nurturing	Parent Behavior Checklist	I
Parental Distress	Parenting Stress Index	I
Parent-Child Dysfunction	Parenting Stress Index	I
Difficult Child	Parenting Stress Index	I
Intensity	Eyberg Child Behavior Inventory	I
Frequency	Eyberg Child Behavior Inventory	I
Problem Behaviors	Behavior Screening Questionnaire	I
Prosocial Behaviors	Behavior Screening Questionnaire	I
Parent Positive Interactions	Dyadic Parent-Child Interaction Coding System (DPCICS)	D (Video)
Parent Negative Interactions	DPCICS	D (Video)
Child Positive Interactions	DPCICS	D (Video)
Child Negative Interactions	DPCICS	D (Video)
Parent Commands	DPCICS	D (Video)
Child Compliance	DPCICS	D (Video)
Child Noncompliance	DPCICS	D (Video)

Lewis et al. study

Variable	Method of Measurement	Directness
SvO_2	Fiber-optic thermodilution pulmonary artery catheter (the Explorer continuous venous oximeter, American Edwards Laboratories, Irvine, Calif)	D

Bruce and Grove study

Variable	Method of Measurement	Directness
Total serum cholesterol	Blood sample	D
LDL	Blood sample	D
HDL	Blood sample	D
Risk level	Calculated from other measures	D

Describing Measures

Carey et al. Study

a. Measure—Dyadic Parent-Child Interaction Coding System (DPCICS)
Developer: Eyberg, Robinson, Kniskern, & O'Brien
Date developed: 1978
Description of method of measurement: A behavioral observational system. Provides codes for parent and child interactional behaviors in 5-minute time blocks. Nine behaviors are coded for mothers (e.g., commands, questions, praise) and eight for the children (e.g., compliance, physical positive, whines). These 17 behaviors were combined into seven variables: parent positives, parent negatives, child positives, child negatives, total commands, total compliant behaviors, and total noncompliant behaviors.
Range of values: Observations of frequency
Critique: Excellent description. Reader has clear understanding of the process of measurement.

b. Measure—The Parent Behavior Checklist (PBC)
Developer: Fox
Date developed: 1994
Range of scores: Not provided
Description of method of measurement: 100-item rating scale developed to measure parenting behaviors and parental expectations of young children between the ages of 1 year and 4 years, 11 months. Normed on an urban population of 1,056 mothers. Measures parenting behaviors on three subscales: (1) discipline measures parental responses to children's challenging behaviors; (2) nurturing measures specific positive parent behaviors that promote a child's psychological growth; and (3) expectations measure parents' developmental expectations. More effective parenting strategies are associated with lower scores on discipline, higher scores on nurturing, and mid-range scores on expectations.
Critique: Good description.

c. Measure—The Parenting Stress Index-Short Form (PSI)
Developer: Abidin
Date developed: 1995
Range of scores: Not provided
Description of method of measurement: A 36-item self-report measure of the amount of stress experienced by parents of young children. Measures parenting stress on three subscales: (1) parent distress measures the amount of distress a parent is experiencing in his or her role as a parent or as a function of personal factors that are related to parenting; (2) parent-child dysfunctional interaction measures the parent's perception that his or her child does not meet the parent's expectations and the interactions with his or her child are not reinforcing; and (3) difficult child measures the basic behavioral characteristics of children that make them either easy or difficult to manage. High scores on any of these subscales are indicative of an increased level of parental stress.
Critique: Clear description of well-developed instrument.

d. Measure—The Eyberg Child Behavior Inventory (ECBI)
Developer: Eyberg & Ross
Date developed: 1978
Range of measures: Not provided.
Description of method of measurement: 36-item inventory that measures behavior problems common to children 2 to 16 years old. An intensity score is determined through the rating of the frequency of each behavior on a scale from 1 (never occurs) to 7 (always occurs). A problem score is determined by having respondents identify each behavior as a current problem with a "yes" or "no" response. The ECBI discriminates between problem and nonproblem children.
Critique: The description of measurement is well done.

e. Measure—The Behavior Screening Questionnaire (BSQ)
Developer: Richman & Graham
Date developed: Original tool published in 1971
Range of measures: Not provided
Description of method of measurement: A screening tool used to identify behavioral and emotional problems in preschool children. For the purposes of this study, the BSQ was adapted to include 12 behavior problem categories common among young children such as sleeping, toileting, and tantrums. New items also were added that assessed prosocial behaviors such as child helps clean up messes, is affectionate, and imitates others.

Lewis et al. Study

a. Measure—SvO_2 (the Explorer continuous venous oximeter)
Developer: American Edwards laboratories, Irvine, California
Date developed: Not given
Description of method of measurement: No description is provided.
Critique: The authors assume this measure is common knowledge. It is not clear from the presentation whether a single value is obtained or whether calculations are made from several measures that are obtained. No explanation is given of the functions of computers in calculating, storing, or displaying the measures.

Bruce and Grove Study

a. Total Serum Cholesterol
The total serum cholesterol value was obtained from the patient's record. No information is provided on the equipment or method used to obtain the value. Since the patients were all receiving care in the same setting, one could expect the procedure and equipment to be consistent across patients and, thus, that values across patients were comparable. However, this is an assumption and is not documented. The authors do report that the National Bureau of Standards and the Centers of Disease Control establish standards that must be followed by laboratories in the measurement and reporting of laboratory values.
b. LDL
The LDL value was obtained from the patient's record. No information is provided on the equipment or method used to obtain the value. Since the patients were all receiving care in the same setting, one could expect the procedure and equipment to be consistent across patients and, thus, that values across patients were comparable. However, this is an assumption and is not documented. The authors do report that the National Bureau of Standards and the Centers of Disease Control establish standards that must be followed by laboratories in the measurement and reporting of laboratory values. The level of LDL was calculated using the following equation: total cholesterol – [HDL cholesterol + triglycerides/5] = LDL
c. HDL
The HDL value was obtained from the patient's record. No information is provided on the equipment or method used to obtain the value. Since the patients were all receiving care in the same setting, one could expect the procedure and equipment to be consistent across patients and, thus, that values across patients were comparable. However, this is an assumption and is not documented. The authors do report that the National Bureau of Standards and the Centers of Disease Control establish standards that must be followed by laboratories in the measurement and reporting of laboratory values.

d. Estimated Cardiovascular Risk Level
The determination of cardiovascular risk level is not discussed in the measurement section of the paper. In the Procedure section, the authors state that each subject was determined to have low, moderate, or high risk for cardiovascular disease. The assessment of cardiac risk was performed by the program nurse in conjunction with the clinic physician and was based on reported risk factors and the results of the serum lipid profile, according to the National Cholesterol Education Program (NCEP) guidelines. The nonlipid risk factors are not defined; however, the description of the sample lists "other reported risk factors" of cigarette smoking, hypertension, obesity, and diagnosed coronary artery disease. How these factors (and perhaps others?) were used to determine the risk level is not explained.

Reliability and Validity of Measures

Carey, Nicholson, and Fox Study

a. Measure—Dyadic Parent-Child Interaction Coding System

Type of Reliability or Validity	Value	From present sample?
Interrater reliability	.85	Yes

b. Measure—The Parent Behavior Checklist

Type of Reliability or Validity	Value	From present sample?
Internal consistency—discipline	.92	No
Internal consistency—nurturing	.91	No
Internal consistency—expectations	.97	No
Test-retest reliability—discipline	.87	No
Test-retest reliability—nurturing	.81	No
Test-retest reliability—expectations	.98	No

c. Measure—The Parenting Stress Index (Short Form)

Type of Reliability or Validity	Value	From present sample?
Test-retest reliability	.84	No
Internal consistency (alpha)	.91	No

d. Measure—The Eyberg Child Behavior Inventory

Type of Reliability or Validity	Value	From present sample?
Test-retest reliability	.86	No
Internal consistency	.98	No

e. Measure—The Behavior Screening Questionnaire

Type of Reliability or Validity	Value	From present sample?
Interrater reliability	.77–.94	No
Correlation between BSQ and clinical rating (concurrent validity)	.88	No

Lewis et al. Study

a. Measure—SvO_2

Type of Reliability or Validity	Value	From present sample?
Correlations between in vivo and in vitro samples	Range = .89 to .97	No
Reliability	Can be used for 102 hours with less than a 1% drift for every 24-hour period	No

Bruce and Grove Study

a. Measure—Total Serum Cholesterol

Type of Reliability or Validity	Value	Present?
Values met the referenced criterion of plus or minus 3% of the true value set by the National Cholesterol Education Program (NCEP)		Yes

b. Measure—LDL

Type of Reliability or Validity	Value	Present?
Values met the referenced criterion of plus or minus 3% of the true value set by the National Cholesterol Education Program (NCEP)		Yes

c. Measure—HDL

Type of Reliability or Validity	Value	Present?
Values met the referenced criterion of plus or minus 3% of the true value set by the National Cholesterol Education Program (NCEP)		Yes

d. Measure—Cardiovascular Risk

Type of Reliability or Validity	Value	Present?
No information provided other than the statement that the classification was based on NCEP guidelines. The fact that the guidelines come from the National Heart, Lung, and Blood Institute of NIH provides some degree of content validity.		

Description of Data Collection Process

Carey et al. Study

"Subjects who met the inclusion criteria were visited in their homes by the first author who reviewed the study procedures and obtained written informed consent. The home visits averaged 1.5 hours in length. Mothers received $50 for participating and their children were given a toy or book. An adapted family form, piloted in previous research . . . was used to obtain family demographic information and to seek maternal responses to questions regarding how parenting was different than expected, whether or not they had attended parenting classes or sought professional help for their child's behavior, and the amount of social support they received for parenting. Next, the child and mother were videotaped playing together with a standard set of safe and age-appropriate toys. A behavioral observational system adapted from the Dyadic Parent-Child Interaction Coding System was followed to structure the videotaping and code the mothers' and children's behaviors. For the first 5 minutes of the videotaped session, the mother was directed to let the child choose an activity and play with the child according to his or her rules. The mother was then directed to choose an activity and play with the child for the next 5 minutes according to the mother's rules. Finally, the mother was instructed to have the child help in cleaning up the play area" (p. 201). After the videotaping, the Parent Behavior Checklist, the Parenting Stress Index-Short Form, The Eyberg Child Behavior Inventory, and The Behavior Screening Questionnaire were administered.

"Each mother was asked the following question during the interview, 'How is parenting (child's name) different from what you expected?' The responses were transcribed by the interviewer at the time of the home visit" (p. 207).

Lewis et al. Study

"After informed consent was obtained and randomization status decided, the patient was left undisturbed for 5 minutes lying supine with the head of the bed elevated 20° to 40°. Baseline SvO_2 was recorded at 1-minute intervals during this 5-minute period (Figure 1). The patient was then turned to the left or right lateral position. A single data collector turned the patient and placed two folded standard pillows, one pillow behind the patient's back and one between the patient's knees. For patients in the delayed-backrub group, SvO_2 was again recorded at 1-minute intervals for 5 minutes after the change in body position. The patient was then given a 1-minute backrub . . . Patients assigned to the immediate-backrub group were turned, and the backrub . . . was given immediately. After the backrub, SvO_2 was measured at 1-minute intervals for 5 minutes. There was then a 5-minute period during which 1-minute measurements were made while the patient remained in the lateral position" (pp. 222-223).

Bruce and Grove Study

The serum lipid values and individual risk factor information were obtained through retrospective medical record review. The greatest threat to the validity of the measures would have been random errors in recording the data from the patient record to a data collection form and then into the computer.

Adequacy of Each Measure

Carey et al. Study

All of the measures in the study have excellent reported reliability from previous studies. Reliability in the present study was not examined except for interrater reliability reported for the DPCICS, which was good. Validity of the instruments was not addressed. All of the instruments used in the study were well established and had been psychometrically developed. One had norm referenced values.

Lewis et al. Study

SvO_2 measured using the Explorer continuous venous oximeter is a reliable and valid measurement method.

Bruce and Grove Study

The measures of lipid levels have acceptable reliability and validity. Although the measure of cardiovascular risk is based on well-accepted guidelines (providing evidence of validity), their application in this study is not sufficiently described to judge reliability. Interrater reliability is not addressed. The authors are not clear about the nonlipid risk factors used in the categorization and the extent to which these are consistent with those recommended by NCEP.

CHAPTER 10—UNDERSTANDING STATISTICS IN RESEARCH

Relevant Terms

Define terms using the glossary in your textbook.

Activities of Data Cleaning

1. Every piece of datum is cross-checked with the original datum for accuracy.
2. All identified errors are corrected.
3. Missing data points are identified.
4. Missing datum is entered into the data file.

Sample Description—You could have listed any three of the following:

1. Estimates of central tendency are calculated for variables relevant to describing the sample.
2. Estimates of dispersion are calculated for variables relevant to describing the sample.
3. Data are examined on each variable using measures of central tendency and dispersion to determine variation in the data and to identify outliers.
4. Relationships among variables relevant to the sample are examined.
5. Differences between groups are examined to demonstrate equivalence of study groups.

Making Connections

Matching Definitions

1. i
2. h
3. f
4. c
5. d
6. e
7. a
8. b
9. g

Matching Categories to Statements

1. b
2. c
3. a
4. d
5. d
6. b
7. d

Significant Differences

1. Partial-bed-rest group distribution

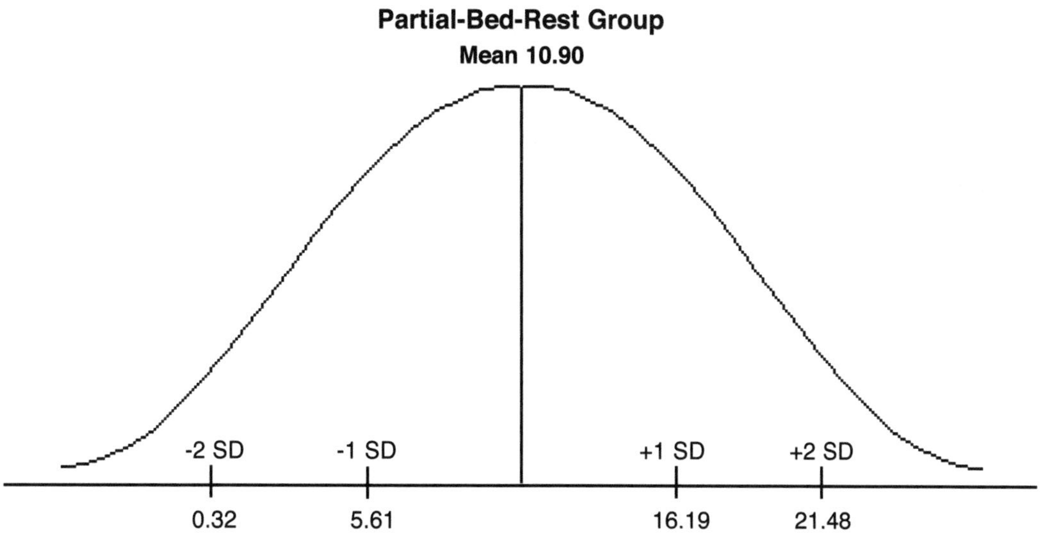

2. Complete-bed-rest group

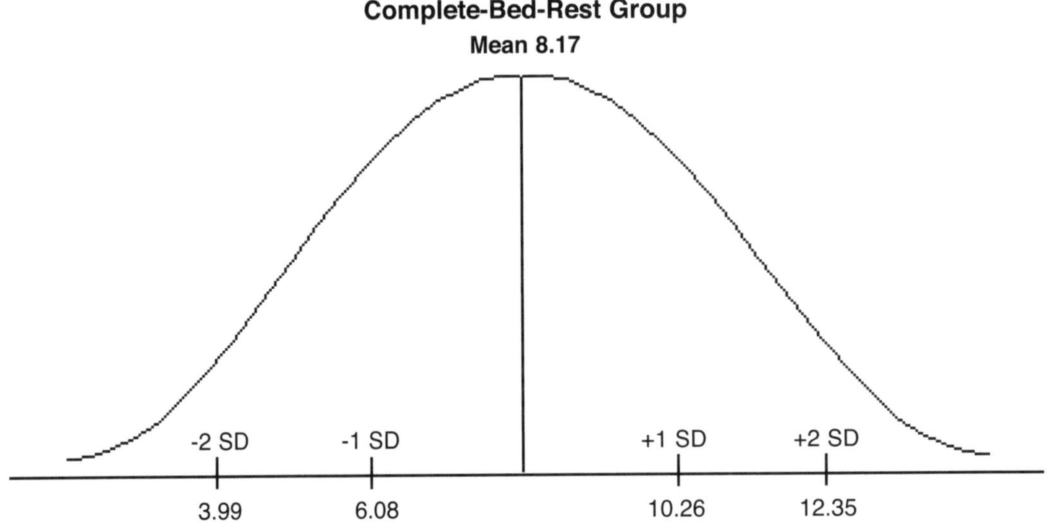

Significance of Results

1. a
2. b
3. a
4. b

Exercises in Critique

1. Variables included in statistical analyses: Bruce and Grove's study

Variable	Level of Measurement
Total serum cholesterol	Interval or higher
LDL	Interval or higher
HDL	Interval or higher
Risk level	Ordinal—treated as nominal

2. Statistical procedures selected by Bruce and Grove to answer their research question.
    1. t-test
    2. McNemar Test for Significance of Changes

3. Groups used in first analysis:
   1. Before participation in the C.A.R.E. program group
   2. After participation in the C.A.R.E. program group
4. These two groups are dependent. The researchers were studying the same subject before and after participation. Refer to discussion of independence and dependence of groups in your textbook.
5. Given that the level of measurement is interval level or higher, and there are two dependent groups (referred to as paired or matched in the figure), the paired (or dependent) t-test is the appropriate statistical test. No other possible statistical tests are identified by this decision tree. The researchers conducted a separate t-test for each variable. Thus, three t-tests were performed. Use of multiple t-tests causes an escalation of the level of significance, increasing the risk of a Type I error (see your textbook). Using analysis of variance, in which all three variables could be included in one analysis followed by posthoc tests to identify the significance of specific variables, might have been a better choice.
6. The variable excluded from the analysis was risk level.
7. Risk level was excluded from the analysis because it is an ordinal level measure and is not an appropriate variable for analysis using a t-test.
8. Mean total cholesterol was reduced by 33.82 mg/dl ($t(194) = -16.76$, $p = 0.00$). The results are significant and predicted.
   The mean LDL level was reduced by 28.97 mg/dl ($t(194) = -15.22$, $p = 0.00$). The results are significant and predicted.
   The mean HDL level was increased by 2.75 mg/dl ($t(194) = 3.27$, $p = 0.001$). The results are significant and predicted.
9. Groups used in Bruce and Grove's second analysis:
   1. Before participation in C.A.R.E group
   2. After participation in C.A.R.E. group
10. According to the decision tree, the recommended analysis for ordinal data is Kruskal-Wallis One-Way Analysis of Variance for Gain Scores. However, the authors treated the risk data as nominal and used the McNemar Test for Significance of Changes. This is a nonparametric analysis that is not described in your textbook. You may find information about it on p. 574 of Burns and Grove (2001). The McNemar test uses the chi square symbol (X^2) as the statistic for the analysis. As a consequence, in a quick examination of the results, it is easy to mistakenly assume that chi square analysis was used.
11. The value obtained from the McNemar test was $X^2 > 98.285$, $p = 0.00$. These results are significant and predicted.
12. Correlation
13. Results of correlational analysis:
    1. Relationship between cardiovascular risk and total cholesterol level ($r = .67$, $p = .000$; 44% variance explained). This means there is a strong and significant correlation between cardiovascular risk and total cholesterol level. The 44%

variance explained is obtained by squaring the r value (r^2) and indicates that 44% of the variation in values of cardiovascular risk and total cholesterol level can be explained by this relationship. However, in considering the meaning of this result, you need to keep in mind that total cholesterol level was used in developing the cardiovascular risk categories. Because of this, the strength of the relationship is overestimated. If one were to remove the effect of total cholesterol level on classifying cardiovascular risk, the amount of relationship between the two variables would be less.

2. Relationship between cardiovascular risk and LDL cholesterol level ($r = .80$, $p = 0.000$; 64% variance explained). This means there is a strong and significant correlation between cardiovascular risk and LDL cholesterol. As in the first relationship discussed, caution is warranted in interpreting this result since LDL cholesterol was used in developing the cardiovascular risk categories and the relationship is probably overestimated.
3. Relationship between cardiovascular risk and HDL cholesterol level ($r = -.12$; 1.5% variance explained). The result is not significant and is unexpected. The authors report that several other studies have found a significant relationship between these two variables. Because HDL was used to develop the risk categories, one would expect to find some degree of relationship between the two variables.

14. Findings:
    1. A significant 13% decrease in the mean total serum cholesterol level occurred after participation in the C.A.R.E. program.
    2. A significant 17% reduction in mean LDL levels occurred after participation in the C.A.R.E. program.
    3. Mean HDL cholesterol levels significantly increased 5.8% after participation in the C.A.R.E. program.
    4. Risk levels were significantly reduced after participation in the C.A.R.E. program. The authors recommend caution in interpreting the results of this analysis. The measurement of risk level in the pretest group was based on the serum lipid profile and the presence of nonlipid risk factors known to affect cardiovascular risk (e.g., exercise, smoking, hypertension, body weight). The measurement of risk level in the posttest group was based only on the serum lipid profile. Other risk factors were not reassessed after participation in the C.A.R.E. program.

    The findings stated by the authors are appropriate in relation to the results. Because a comparative descriptive design was used, it is not possible to state that the C.A.R.E. program caused the results. A quasi-experimental design with a comparison or control group would be needed to make that claim. Without a control group, the inference that the program caused the results is unwarranted since there is insufficient evidence that the changes would not have occurred if the program had not been provided.

15. Strengths and weaknesses of statistical analyses:
The t-test was appropriate given the level of measurement of the variables. The selection of another analysis strategy such as ANOVA might have reduced the risk for a Type I error from escalation of the level of significance due to the use of repeated t-tests. The use of the McNemar test was acceptable given the level of measurement. Difficulties in interpreting results were due to problems related to design and measurement, not to the statistical procedures used.
16. Conclusions:
"The findings may demonstrate an association between the C.A.R.E. program and the improvements in serum lipid values for the sample."
17. The authors are careful to qualify their conclusion by indicating that the findings may demonstrate an association. This statement is warranted by the data.
18. Implications
    1. "The results do support the use of educational programs in addition to risk factor assessment in reducing cardiac risk levels."
    2. "Education can be effective in improving lipid profiles and potentially decrease the incidence of CAD (coronary artery disease)."
    3. "Decreasing risk for CAD and the associated loss of productivity, disability, and death could enhance quality of life."
19. Evaluation of implications:
The authors walk a narrow line in discussing the implications of their findings while avoiding the assertion that the educational program caused the changes they found. The important implication is that there is sufficient evidence that the educational program was effective in reducing risk to warrant quasi-experimental studies to test the cause-effect relationship.
20. Clinical significance:
"This study demonstrates that nurse-managed health education programs such as the C.A.R.E. program can have dramatic impact on individuals' health and can potentially improve quality of life for high-risk populations."
21. Generalizations:
    1. Educational programs in general
    2. Nurse-managed health education programs
22. Suggestions for further studies:
    1. Quasi-experimental studies
    2. Longitudinal studies
    3. Studies using different populations such as minorities, women, children, and the elderly
    4. Cost-benefit analyses

CHAPTER 11—INTRODUCTION TO QUALITATIVE RESEARCH

Relevant Terms

Define terms using the glossary in your textbook.

Making Connections

Matching Characteristics with Type of Research

1. b
2. a
3. b
4. b
5. a
6. b
7. a
8. b
9. a
10. a

Characteristics of Rigor in Qualitative Research

1. Openness
2. Scrupulous adherence to a philosophical perspective
3. Thoroughness in collecting data
4. Consideration of all of the data in the subjective theory development phase

Characteristics of Researcher-Participant Relationships in Qualitative Research

1. The researcher influences the individuals being studied and, in turn, is influenced by them.
2. The mere presence of the researcher may alter behavior in the setting.
3. The researcher's personality is a key factor in conducting the study.
4. The researcher needs to become closely involved in the subject's experience in order to interpret it.
5. It is necessary for the researcher to be open to the perceptions of the participants, rather than to attach his or her own meaning to the experience.
6. Individuals being studied often participate in determining research questions, guiding data collection, and interpreting results.

Methods of Reducing Data in Qualitative Research

1. Coding—developing categories
2. Reflective remarks
3. Marginal remarks
4. Memoing
5. Developing propositions

Methods of Drawing Conclusions

1. Counting
2. Noting patterns, themes
3. Seeing plausibility
4. Clustering
5. Making metaphors
6. Splitting variables
7. Subsuming particulars into the general
8. Factoring
9. Noting relations between variables
10. Finding intervening variables
11. Building a logical chain of evidence
12. Making conceptual/theoretical coherence

Matching Qualitative Method with Characteristics

1. c
2. b
3. a
4. c
5. a
6. d
7. c
8. b
9. d
10. a

Storytelling

Do the storytelling exercise and discuss your findings with your faculty.

Stages of Qualitative Data Analysis

1. Description
2. Analysis
3. Interpretation

Exercises in Critique

1. An exploratory analysis was conducted on the interview data. Separate themes were developed for each mother. These themes were then merged into two sets, one for mothers of children with CHD and another for mothers of healthy children.
2. Mothers of children with CHD:
    - The unexpected
    - Vigilance
    - Uncertainty
    - Positive outlook

   Mothers of healthy children:
    - Temperament
    - Strains
    - Rewards
    - Expectations
    - Discipline
    - Comparisons
3. Supportive data, in the form of maternal quotes, were anchored to the common themes. Two independent reviewers provided content validation by reviewing the emerging themes and supportive interview data.
4. Qualitative analyses of mothers' responses to the question of how their parenting was different from what they expected it to be resulted in a very different picture emerging for mothers of children with CHD compared with mothers of healthy children. This discovery would not have been possible without the qualitative data and provided rich information regarding the parenting experience.
5. The authors recommend providing time for families to tell their stories. This allows the nurse to understand the lived experience of parenting a child with congenital heart disease. Mothers need to tell stories and share their personal experience of parenting even when they have healthy children. This information can be helpful to the nurse in designing strategies to support families during this life experience.

CHAPTER 12—CRITIQUING NURSING STUDIES

Relevant Terms

1. i
2. c
3. a
4. j
5. g
6. b
7. e
8. h
9. f
10. d

Key Ideas

1. strengths, weaknesses, meaning, and significance
2. You might include any three of the following:
   a. What are the major strengths of the study?
   b. What are the major weaknesses of the study?
   c. Are the findings from the study an accurate reflection of reality?
   d. What is the significance of the findings for nursing?
   e. Are the findings consistent with those for previous studies?
3. You might critique research to share the findings with another health care professional. You might read and critique studies to solve a problem in practice or to summarize research in a topic area for use in practice. You might critique a proposed study to determine whether it is ethical to conduct in your clinical agency.
4. comprehension, comparison, analysis, and evaluation
5. a. Descriptive vividness
   b. Methodological congruence
   c. Analytical preciseness
   d. Theoretical connectedness
   e. Heuristic relevance

Exercises in Critique

Conduct the critiques of the studies included in Appendix B of this study guide. Review the answers for the critique exercises for Chapters 3 through 10 to assist you in these critiques. Also ask your instructor to clarify any questions that you might have.

CHAPTER 13—USING RESEARCH IN NURSING PRACTICE

Relevant Terms

1. e
2. g
3. f
4. a
5. c
6. h
7. d
8. b

Key Ideas

1. Research utilization promotes desired outcomes for patients, nurses, and health care agencies. Some of these positive outcomes are identified below.
   a. Improve patients' outcomes such as decreased signs and symptoms of illness, increased function, decreased recovery time, decreased length of hospitalization, increased return-to-work rate, increased satisfaction with care, increased health promotion and illness prevention behaviors.
   b. Improve the quality of care
   c. Decrease the cost of care
   d. Improve the work environment for nurses and promote nurses' productivity.
   e. Provide increased access to care by providing different types of health care agencies and services by a variety of health care providers.
2. Obtain the answers to these questions by gathering information in the agency where you are doing your clinical hours this semester. Ask your faculty if these questions might be covered in class.
3. You might identify any of the following:
   a. Research journals (online or paper copy)
   b. Clinical journals with a major focus on publishing research articles
   c. Nursing research conferences
   d. Professional nursing meetings and conferences
   e. Some collaborative groups of nurses and other health professionals that share research findings
   f. Television news reports
   g. Newspapers
   h. Some popular magazines
   i. Web sites with national research-based guidelines
   j. Agency research newsletters
4. You might identify any of the following:
   a. Axford and Cutchen (1977) developed a preoperative teaching program.
   b. Dracup and Breu (1978) devised a care plan for grieving spouses.
   c. Wichita (1977) developed a program to treat and prevent constipation in nursing home residents.

5. a. Identification and synthesis of multiple studies on a selected topic.
   b. Organization of research knowledge into a solution or clinical protocol for practice.
   c. Transformation of the clinical protocol into specific nursing actions that are administered to patients.
   d. Clinical evaluation of the new practice to determine whether it produced the desired outcome.
6. You might identify any of the following:
   a. Structured preoperative teaching
   b. Reducing diarrhea in tube-fed patients
   c. Preoperative sensory preparation to promote recovery
   d. Preventing decubitus ulcers
   e. Intravenous cannula change
   f. Closed urinary drainage systems
   g. Distress reduction through sensory preparation
   h. Mutual goal setting in patient care
   i. Clean intermittent catheterization
   j. Pain: deliberative nursing interventions
7. a. Researcher-generated reports and findings have barriers. Examples: Limited research conducted for certain clinical problems; studies conducted lack replication; limited communication of research findings; research reports are complex and difficult to read.
   b. Barriers created by practicing nurses. Examples: Practicing nurses do not value research; they are unwilling to read research reports; they lack the skills to read research reports; they have limited desire to change practice base on research.
   c. Barriers created by organizations. Examples: Some organizations have traditional leadership that is reluctant to change; some organizations do not value research and do not provide support for making changes based on research.
8. You might include any of the following:
   a. Previous practice
   b. Felt needs/problems
   c. Innovativeness
   d. Norms of the social system
9. a. Relative advantage
   b. Compatibility
   c. Complexity
   d. Trialability
   e. Observability
10. examining the innovation or change for practice and then deciding not to adopt it
11. that the innovation was never seriously considered for use in practice

12. a. Direct application. Description: occurs when an innovation is used exactly as it was developed.
    b. Reinvention. Description: occurs when adopters modify the innovation to meet their own needs.
    c. Indirect effects. Description: occur when nurses incorporate research findings into their knowledge base and use this information to defend a point or to write agency protocols or policies or a clinical paper.
13. a. Replacement discontinuance
    b. Disenchantment discontinuance
14. a. Published integrative reviews of research
    b. Published meta-analysis
15. current best
16. researchers, clinicians, and theorists
17. a. National clinical practice guidelines or standards
    b. Published research-based protocols, algorithms, or clinical pathways
    c. Summary of current studies, integrative review, and meta-analysis that are used to develop a protocol or algorithm for use in practice
18. evidenced-based
19. identified standard that an agency wants to achieve in patient care, such as having a 1% complication rate for IM injections
20. clearly developed steps for implementing a treatment or intervention in practice (These steps are documented with research findings.)
21. a. Agency for Healthcare Research and Quality (AHRQ) http://www.ahrq.gov/clinic/epc/
    b. National Guideline Clearinghouse (NGC) http://www.guideline.gov/

Making Connections

1. e
2. c
3. a
4. d
5. b

appendix B Published Studies

MATERNAL FACTORS RELATED TO PARENTING YOUNG CHILDREN WITH CONGENITAL HEART DISEASE

LYNN K. CAREY, BONNIE C. NICHOLSON, ROBERT A. FOX

Abstract

The purpose of this study was to compare the early child-rearing practices between mothers of young children with congenital heart disease (CHD) and mothers of healthy children. In addition, maternal stress, parental developmental expectations, and the early behavioral and emotional development of their children were explored. Maccoby's (1992) socialization theory emphasizing the reciprocal nature of mother-child interactions provided the framework for this study. Findings from quantitative self-report measures and videotaped parent-child interactions showed a remarkable similarity between mothers of children with CHD and mothers of healthy children. In contrast, qualitative data revealed important differences with mothers of CHD children reporting high levels of vigilance with their children. The important role of promoting the principle of normalization among mothers of children with CHD and ensuring a sufficient support system is discussed.

PARENTS AND OTHER SIGNIFICANT CAREGIVERS play an important role in children's development (Collins, Maccoby, Steinberg, Hetherington, & Bornstein, 2000). There are numerous factors that influence the quality of parenting that children receive (Belsky, 1990). The health status of a child, including the onset of a chronic illness, is one of many factors that can contribute to the quality of child rearing (Kazak, 1989). When considering that up to 30% of children have a chronic health condition (Newacheck & Halfon, 1998), 11% of whom are living with conditions considered moderate to severe (Newacheck, Stoddard, & McManus, 1993), a significant number of families are faced with an even more challenging future than they had anticipated. How parents respond to this situation can affect both the short- and long-term developmental outcomes for their children.

Conceptual model

The family context is an important contributing factor in the socialization of children (Maccoby & Martin, 1983). More specifically, the role of parents in influencing their children's outcomes has increasingly been the focus of research. What has emerged is

From Carey, L.K., Nicholson, B.C., & Fox, R.A. (2002). Maternal factors related to parenting young children with congenital heart disease. *Journal of Pediatric Nursing, 17*(3), 174–183.

the general finding that parents and children influence each other in a reciprocal manner (Maccoby, 1992). For example, children who have difficult temperaments are likely to bring out different responses in their parents than children who are more easygoing. Similarly, children born with significant health impairments may also elicit unique parental responses (e.g., overprotective). How parents respond over time can influence the children's short- and long-term developmental outcomes. In general, an authoritative parenting style (i.e., parents who are responsive to their children's needs and set reasonable limits on their behavior) produces the most favorable childhood outcomes (Steinberg, Lamborn, Darling, Mounts, & Dornbusch, 1994).

There are multiple determinants that impact parenting practices (Belsky, 1990), including socioeconomic and maternal factors. For example, Fox, Platz, and Bentley (1995) reported less favorable parenting practices among mothers who were younger, single, from lower income and educational levels, and who had more than one child living at home. Numerous other factors including marital satisfaction, level of spousal support, and the mental health of the parent can influence child-rearing practices (Simons, Beamon, Conger, & Chao, 1993). In addition, the child's unique characteristics, including temperament (O'Conner, Deater-Deckard, Fulker, Rutter, & Plomin, 1998) and health status (Dolgin, Phipps, & Harrow, 1990) also influence parenting practices. Regarding the rearing of chronically ill children, Maccoby's (1992) model would predict that parents may significantly alter their child-rearing patterns to accommodate these children's special needs. In fact, Van Dongen-Melmen and Sanders-Woudstra (1986) suggested that it would be difficult to imagine parents who would not be at least somewhat overly protective of their children. This overprotective parenting style, fueled at least in part by parental anxiety, could hamper the overall development of these children (Utens et al., 1994).

Purpose

The purpose of this study was to compare the early child-rearing practices between mothers of children with congenital heart disease (CHD) and mothers of healthy children. In addition, parenting stress, parental expectations of their young children, and the early behavioral and emotional development of toddlers and preschoolers were explored.

Review of the literature

Parents often respond with shock and disbelief when a diagnosis of a chronic illness in their child is first made (Sabbeth, 1984). Parenting a child with a chronic illness has been considered to be a highly stressful, demanding experience for the parents and family (Austin, 1991). However, positive adaptation and growth has also been reported among these families (Clawson, 1996).

Most available studies regarding the parenting of children with CHD have emphasized parental adjustment to the diagnosis (Emery, 1989), the demands and related stress that these children place on the family (Svavarstottir & McCubbin, 1996), and early care-giving issues, particularly infant feeding difficulties (Lobo, 1992). Relatively less attention has been devoted to the emotional adjustment of these children (DeMaso, Beardslee, Silbert, & Fyler, 1991). Goldberg, Simmons, Newman, Campbell, and Fowler (1991) studied mother-infant interactions in mothers of children with CHD and mothers of healthy children. Maternal-child attachments in the CHD group were less secure than attachments in the healthy group. In the CHD group, securely attached infants showed greater improvement in their physical health than those infants who were less securely attached. DeMaso, et al. (1990) found that the behavioral adjustment of children with CHD was significantly related to the level of parenting stress.

With recent medical advances significantly improving the prognosis for children with CHD (Marino & Lipshitz, 1991), the concept of normalization (Krulik, 1980) has been extended to these families. Normalization is described as "the constant process of actively accommodating the changing physical and emotional needs of the child" (Deatrick, Knafl, & Walsh, 1988, p. 17). To accomplish normalization in families of children with chronic illnesses, health care professionals commonly advise these parents to raise their children as close to normal as possible (Deatrick, Knafl, & Murphy-Moore, 1999). This normalization philosophy is intended to minimize the impact of a chronic health condition and optimize the child's normative development while fostering a greater acceptance of the child with a chronic illness within society (Holaday, 1984).

Methodology

Two groups of mothers with children between 2 and 5 years of age from a large urban area in the Midwest made up the study sample. The first group included mothers of children with moderate to severe CHD, recruited through a large pediatric cardiology clinic at a children's hospital. Cardiac severity was rated by each child's pediatric cardiologist using the Cardiologist's Perception of Medical Severity (DeMaso, et al., 1991), which has a rating scale ranging from 1 = insignificant (disorder has no impact on child's health) to 5 = severe (uncorrectable lesion or only complex, palliative repair possible), and an inter-rater reliability of .97. Five pediatric cardiologists participated in this study. Subjects in the CHD group required a severity rating of at least moderate (3 or higher) to be included in this study. The second group included mothers of healthy children (absence of chronic illnesses, significant health conditions, or birth anomalies) who were recruited from pediatric medical practices and school settings and matched with the first group on the child's age and gender and maternal marital and socioeconomic status.

Subjects who met the inclusion criteria were visited in their homes by the first author who reviewed the study procedures and obtained written informed consent. The home visits averaged about 1.5 hours in length. Mothers received $50 for participating and their children were given a toy or book.

An adapted family form, piloted in previous research (Nicholson, Anderson, Fox, & Brenner, in press), was used to obtain family demographic information and to seek maternal responses to questions regarding how parenting was different than expected, whether or not they had attended parenting classes or sought professional help for their child's behavior, and the amount of social support they received for parenting. Next, the child and mother were videotaped playing together with a standard set of safe and age appropriate toys. A behavioral observational system adapted from the Dyadic Parent-Child Interaction Coding System (DPCICS; Eyberg, Robinson, Kniskern, & O'Brien, 1978) was followed to structure the videotaping and code the mothers' and children's behaviors. For the first 5 minutes of the videotaped session, the mother was directed to let the child choose an activity and play with the child according to his or her rules. The mother was then directed to choose an activity and play with the child for the next 5 minutes according to the mother's rules. Finally, the mother was instructed to have the child help in cleaning up the play area.

After the videotaping, the instruments described below were administered. The Parent Behavior Checklist (PBC; Fox, 1994) is a 100-item rating scale developed to measure parenting behaviors and parental expectations of young children between the ages of 1 year and 4 years, 11 months. Normed on an urban population of 1,056 mothers, the PBC measures parenting behaviors on three subscales: (1) *discipline* measures parental responses to children's challenging behaviors (e.g., "When my child has a temper tantrum, I spank him or her"), (2) *nurturing* measures specific positive parent behaviors that promote a child's psychological growth (e.g., "I praise my child for learning new things"), and (3) *expectations* measures parents' developmental expectations (e.g., "My child should be old enough to share toys"). More effective parenting strategies are associated with lower scores on discipline, higher scores on nurturing, and mid-range scores on expectations. Internal consistencies and test-retest reliabilities for each subscale, respectively, are as follows: discipline = .92, .87; nurturing = .91, .81; and expectations = .97, .98. The PBC was selected for this study to assess the parental expectations and reported parenting practices of the families of children with CHD.

The Parenting Stress Index-Short Form (PSI) is a 36-item, self-report measure of the amount of stress experienced by parents of young children (Abidin, 1995). The PSI measures parenting stress on three subscales: (1) *parent distress* measures the amount of distress a parent is experiencing in his or her role as a parent or as a function of personal factors that are related to parenting; (2) *parent-child dysfunctional interaction* measures the parent's perception that his or her child does not meet the parent's expectations and the interactions with his or her child are not reinforcing; and (3) *difficult child* measures the basic behavioral characteristics of children that make them either easy or difficult to manage. High scores on any of these subscales are indicative of an increased level of parental stress. Test-retest and alpha reliabilities for the PSI total score are .84 and .91, respectively. This measure was selected to detect potential parental stress related to rearing a child with CHD. The Eyberg Child Behavior Inventory (ECBI; Eyberg & Ross, 1978) is a 36-item inventory that measures behavior problems common to children 2 to 16 years old. An intensity score is determined through the rating of the frequency of each behavior on a scale from 1 (never occurs) to 7 (always occurs). A problem score is determined by having respondents identify each behavior as a current problem with a "yes" or "no" response. The ECBI discriminates between problem and nonproblem children (Robinson, Eyberg, & Ross, 1980). Reliabilities of this scale range from .86 (test-retest) to .98 (internal consistency). The Behavior Screening Questionnaire (BSQ; Richman & Graham, 1971) is a screening tool used to identify behavioral and emotional problems in preschool children. Inter-rater reliabilities are reported between .77 and .94. A correlation of .88 between the BSQ and clinical rating of 3-year-old children has been reported. For the purposes of this study, the BSQ was adapted to include 12 behavior problem categories common among young children such as sleeping, toileting, and tantrums. New items also were added that assessed prosocial behaviors such as child helps clean up messes, is affectionate, and imitates others. The ECBI and BSQ were selected for this study to assess the present level of behavioral development of children with CHD.

Results

A total of 39 prospective mothers of children with CHD met the study's criteria and could be contacted by phone or mail. Mothers were contacted consecutively until a sample size of 30 was reached. Six subjects could not participate due to personal reasons (e.g., moving, caring for a seriously ill parent). The sample of 30 mothers of healthy children was matched with the CHD sample based on the children's age and gender and maternal marital and socioeconomic status.

For the CHD group, children's mean age was 3.44 years (SD = 0.93), mothers' mean age was 33.5 years (SD = 4.45), and the family included an average of 2.03 children (range = 1-5). For the healthy group, children's mean age was 3.43 years (SD = 0.94), mothers' mean age was 32.13 years (SD = 4.16), and the family included an average of 2.20 children (range = 1-4). Additional demographic data for both study groups are shown in Table 1.

Table 1. Demographic characteristics of families by study group

	Congenital Heart Disease		Healthy	
Variable	**n**	**%**	**n**	**%**
Marital status				
Married	25	83.4	25	83.4
Not married	5	16.6	5	16.6
Mother's education				
High school or less	7	23.3	5	16.7
Beyond high school	23	76.7	25	83.3
Father's education				
High school or less	12	40.0	9	30.0
Beyond high school	18	60.0	21	70.0
Mother's employment				
Homemaker	11	36.7	5	16.7
Working outside home	19	63.3	25	83.3
Father's employment				
Professional	10	33.3	14	48.3
Nonprofessional	20	66.6	15	51.7
Family income				
$50,000 or less	17	56.7	11	36.7
More than $50,000	13	43.3	19	63.3
Children's gender				
Male	17	56.6	17	56.6
Female	13	43.3	13	43.3
Children's ethnicity				
African American	4	13.3	4	13.3
Caucasian	25	83.3	25	83.3
Biracial	1	3.3	1	3.3
Birth order				
First	7	23.3	10	33.3
Middle	1	3.3	5	16.7
Last	12	40.0	13	43.3
Only	10	33.3	2	6.7
Parenting classes				
Yes	7	23.3	6	20.0
No	23	76.7	24	80.0
Amount of social support				
Low	1	3.3	4	13.3
Medium	6	20.0	10	33.4
High	23	76.7	16	53.3

Chi-square analyses found a significant difference between the groups on maternal employment (p = .045) with more mothers of children with CHD as full-time homemakers (36.7%) than mothers of healthy children (16.7%).

Analyses of additional demographic variables including maternal age, child age, child gender, number of children in the family, and mother's and father's number of hours working outside of the home, family socioeconomic status (based on main wage earner's occupation), and maternal marital status showed no differences between groups (all $p > .05$). There was a trend ($p < .058$) for mothers of children with CHD to report higher levels of social support for their parenting (76.7%) compared to mothers of healthy children (53.3%). None of the families had sought professional help for their children's behavior. Additional characteristics of the CHD sample are shown in Table 2.

Table 2. Health-related characteristics of children with congenital heart disease

Variable	n	%	M	SD*	Range
Time of diagnosis					
Fetal diagnosis	2	6.7			
At birth	14	46.7			
First month of life	10	33.3			
After first month of life	4	13.3			
Cardiologists' perception of medical severity					
3-Moderate	2	6.7			
4-Marked	20	66.6			
5-Severe	8	26.7			
Total hospitalizations			2.37	1.15	0-5
Total days in hospital			30.57	22.10	0-106
Cardiac operations			2.10	1.15	0-5
Cardiac catherizations			1.57	1.16	0-5
Outpatient visits since diagnosis			12.50	4.82	4-28

*SD = Standard deviation

For the CHD group, all of the children had been diagnosed by nine months of age, with most diagnosed within the first month of life (86.7%). Tetralogy of Fallot was the most common diagnosis ($n = 6$), followed by hypoplastic left heart syndrome ($n = 4$) and aortic stenosis ($n = 2$); the remaining diagnoses were unique to particular children in the sample (e.g., bicuspid aortic valve and mild aortic stenosis; tricuspid atresia; ventricular septal defect). Of the sample, 46.7% were taking cardiac medications, although none of the children's activities were restricted at the time of this study.

Self-report parenting and child behavior measures

A series of analyses were computed with group assignment as the independent variable (CHD, healthy) and the scores on the self-report measures as the dependent variables. Scores that were conceptually related were analyzed together using multivariate analyses of variance (MANOVA); other scores were analyzed using one-way, analyses of variance (ANOVA). Significant MANOVAs were followed up with univariate *F* tests. Mothers' scores on the four self-report measures are shown by group in Table 3.

Table 3. Summary scores for self-report measures by study group

	Congenital Heart Disease		Healthy	
Variable	**M**	**SD***	**M**	**SD***
Parent behavior checklist				
Expectations	45.16	9.99	50.53	9.56
Discipline	40.43	10.02	42.43	7.91
Nurturing	55.53	11.78	56.03	11.48
Parenting stress index				
Parental distress	26.00	6.65	24.77	8.50
Parent-child dysfunction	18.10	5.98	16.77	4.21
Difficult child	26.50	6.38	26.03	8.07
Eyberg child behavior inventory				
Intensity	100.17	28.69	99.13	25.59
Frequency	10.30	16.70	9.20	12.61
Behavior screening questionnaire				
Problem behaviors	23.13	4.40	21.77	3.65
Prosocial behaviors	44.17	5.12	44.20	4.48

*SD = Standard deviation

A MANOVA was computed with the discipline and nurturing subscales of the PBC. No significant differences were found between mothers of children with CHD and mothers of healthy children ($p = .69$). Based on an ANOVA, a significant difference between groups was found for the expectations scores on the PBC [$F\ (1,58) = 4.51$, $p = .038$). As shown in Table 3, mothers of children with CHD had significantly lower expectations than mothers of healthy children. A MANOVA was computed for the three subscale scores of the Parenting Stress Index; no significant effect was found ($p = .75$). A MANOVA including the two subscales of the ECBI and the problem behavior subscale of the BSQ was not significant ($p = .42$). A final ANOVA with the prosocial behavior subscale of the BSQ also was not significant ($p = .30$).

Videotaped parent-child interactions

Coding of the videotaped parent-child interaction was completed using an adapted version of the DPCICS (Eyberg, et al., 1994). This system allows observers to rate the frequency of selected behaviors for both the child and the mother in 5-minute time blocks. For the present study, nine behaviors were measured for the mothers (e.g., commands, questions, praise) and eight for the children (e.g., compliance, physical positive, whines). To remove the effects of observer bias, an individual trained and experienced in using the coding system coded the videotapes. This individual had already achieved high interobserver reliability for this observation measure, being trained to an 80% agreement criterion using other videotapes of parent-child interactions. A second trained observer rated one third (20) of the tapes to obtain an estimate of interobserver reliability. A Pearson correlation was computed between observers for each of the mother and child behaviors combined across the three phases of the directed interaction (child directed play, parent directed play, and clean up); the average inter-rater reliability coefficient was .85.

For purposes of data analyses, the 17 separate mother and child behaviors were combined across the three observations (child directed play, parent directed play, and clean up) into the following seven variables: *parent positives* (total number of questions, praise, and physical positives expressed by the mother); *parent negatives* (total criticisms, yells, whines, physical negatives, and destructive behaviors by the mother); *child positives* (physical positive behaviors by the child); *child negatives* (total number of criticism, yells, whines, physical negative behaviors, and destructive behaviors by the child); *total commands* by the mother; *total compliant behaviors* by the child; and *total noncompliant behaviors* by the child. This combination of separate variables was necessary because of some variables yielding zero frequencies during the videotaped observation (e.g., parent yells, parent physical negative behaviors, destructive child behaviors). The combined behavioral frequencies are shown in Table 4.

A series of analyses were computed on these variables. A MANOVA with group assignment (mothers of children with CHD, mothers of healthy children) as the independent variable, and parent positives and child positives as the dependent variables, was not significant ($p = .37$). A second MANOVA with two dependent variables, parent negatives and child negatives, also was not significant ($p = .41$). Separate ANOVAs were computed and no significant differences were found between mothers of children with CHD and mothers of healthy children for parent commands ($p = .60$), child compliance ($p = .49$), and child noncompliance ($p = .65$). An additional analysis was done by computing a child's compliance percentage (compliance percentage = child compliance behaviors/parent commands x 100). The compliance percentage for children with CHD ($M = 67\%$, $SD = 21\%$) did not differ significantly ($p = .82$) from healthy children ($M = 68\%$, $SD = 19\%$).

Table 4. Combined maternal and child behaviors from videotaped interactions

	Congenital Heart Disease		Healthy	
Variable	**M**	**SD***	**M**	**SD***
Parent positive	60.13	4.98	59.53	4.98
Parent negative	1.83	0.49	0.93	0.49
Child positive	0.00	0.03	0.06	0.03
Child negative	2.77	1.03	2.07	1.03
Parent commands	27.97	3.12	25.67	3.12
Child compliance	17.30	1.64	15.70	1.64
Child noncompliance	7.00	1.41	6.10	1.41

*SD = Standard deviation

Qualitative parenting responses

Each mother was asked the following question during the interview: "How is parenting (child's name) different from what you expected?" The responses were transcribed by the interviewer at the time of the home visit. An exploratory content analysis was conducted on the interview data, and themes for each of the separate interviews were identified. All themes were reviewed separately for mothers of children with CHD and mothers of healthy children; common themes for each of the groups were delineated. Supportive data, in the form of maternal quotes, were anchored to the common themes. Two independent reviewers provided content validation by reviewing the emerging themes and supportive interview data. Final content themes revisions were made. The most frequently endorsed themes and the supporting interview statements for each group of mothers are shown in Table 5.

Table 5. Most frequently endorsed interview themes and supporting statements for mothers of children with congenital heart disease (CHD) and mothers of healthy children

Interview Theme	Number of Respondents	Supporting Maternal Statements
Mothers of Children with CHD		
(1) The unexpected	19	We didn't learn about his condition until he was 1½ weeks. Then we found out about his heart and it was a complete shock.
(2) Vigilance	19	We are not comfortable leaving her overnight. I have not slept away from my kids for 4 years.
(3) Uncertainty	19	He sleeps with us each night. I am afraid he will stop breathing. There is always that fear.
(4) Positive outlook	14	We try to live each day fuller now; we don't take a day for granted.
(5) Normalization	11	I would say I do not treat him differently. Just make sure he gets his medicine. I watch his activity level, if he is out of breath or turning blue. Otherwise, I treat him like a normal kid; he is a normal kid.
(6) Stress	10	It's a lot more stressful on the whole family. I feel bad for our older daughter. I think she had to grow up fast.
Mothers of Healthy Children		
(1) Temperament	22	He has a strong personality and he will keep asking until we give in.
(2) Strains	13	I always thought it (parenting) would be a lot of work and it is. But I am surprised at the amount of energy it takes.
(3) Rewards	11	I knew we would enjoy parenthood, but I didn't realize all the rewards and special times that go along with it.
(4) Expectations	9	Hardest job on earth. It really is; nothing could have prepared me for it.
(5) Discipline	9	I didn't expect to feel inadequate, not knowing if I am doing the right thing. Like when I discipline her.
(6) Comparisons	7	I can compare him with my other child. He is much more active and independent.

In addition to these themes, seven or more mothers of children with CHD reported using differential discipline, being concerned about comments from other parents with healthy children, feeding issues, and the children's unique temperaments. One additional theme generated by mothers of healthy children was the difficulties of balancing home and work.

Discussion

The purpose of this study was to compare the parenting practices of mothers of children with CHD and mothers of healthy children. With the exception of more mothers of children with CHD being full-time homemakers ($n = 11$) compared to mothers of healthy children ($n = 5$), these two groups were highly similar on several maternal, child, and family factors known to influence child rearing, including mother's age and marital status, child's age and gender, and family's socioeconomic status. Consequently, the only important variable that distinguished the two groups was the presence or absence of child with CHD.

What emerged from the analyses of quantitative data obtained from the maternal self-report inventories and the coded, videotaped mother-child interactions were the remarkable similarities between mothers of children with CHD and mothers of healthy children. Both maternal groups reported similar nurturing and discipline practices with their young children. In addition, the parent stress levels related to child rearing did not differ between groups. These self-report findings were further validated by the videotaped parent-child interactions. Despite coding 17 different maternal and child behaviors, no significant differences for any of these behaviors were found between the two groups of mothers and their children. In fact, the only significant difference that was found between groups was that mothers of children with CHD had lower expectations for their children than mothers of healthy children. This difference in expectations also has been reported between mothers of mildly handicapped and nonhandicapped preschoolers (Tucker & Fox, 1995). However, when interpreting this difference for the present study, it is important to note that the mean expectations scores for both groups were well within one standard deviation of the mean and thus could be considered as "normal" developmental expectations. The outcomes for the children also were similar. Children with CHD did not differ from healthy children in terms of the frequencies of their challenging or prosocial behaviors.

These findings are surprising and would have been difficult to predict based on the study's conceptual model, namely that parents and children influence each other in a reciprocal manner (Maccoby, 1992). The literature (Davis, Brown, & Campbell, 1998) clearly shows that mothers of children with CHD experience high levels of daily stress. In response to this difficult situation, this study's conceptual model would predict that these mothers should be more likely to engage in an overly protective and more permissive parenting style than mothers of healthy children. Yet with the exception of parental expectations, which were lower for mothers of children with CHD, these two groups of mothers appeared very similar in their parenting practices and in their experiences of parental stress related to childrearing issues. Moreover, the outcomes for their children's social-emotional development, based on the frequency of reported and observed challenging and prosocial behaviors, were unexpected. Based on our conceptual model, had we been correct in predicting a permissive parenting style among mothers with children with CHD, it would have followed that there would be less positive outcomes for their children (Brenner & Fox, 1999). However, based on the present data, children with CHD could not be distinguished from healthy children by their behavior.

Perhaps for this group of mothers with children with CHD, the normalization advice they received from the health care professionals had a beneficial impact on their child rearing. Based on interviews with members of the health care team, the pediatric cardiology clinic fully embraces the concept of normalization for its families. The concept of "treat your child normally" is routinely communicated to families by physicians and the nursing staff (see Moller, Neal, & Hoffman, 1988). However, we did not collect specific data on the level of normalization advice provided to each mother or on their ability to understand and apply this principle with their children. Also, there was a range of responses on the self-report measures suggesting that some mothers of CHD children may have applied normalization strategies better than others. This conclusion is supported by recent research that suggests a continuum of family management strategies in response to a child's chronic illness ranging from thriving to floundering (Knafl, Breitmayer, Gallo, & Zoeller, 1996).

The quantitative data collected in the present study does not tell the whole story. Mothers in both groups were asked how their parenting was different from what they had expected it to be. Qualitative analyses of their responses to this question resulted in a very different picture emerging for mothers of children with CHD compared to mothers of healthy children. These mothers did not expect to have a child with a serious health condition and were experiencing significant uncertainty regarding their child's future. These mothers responded to this situation by maintaining heightened levels of vigilance regarding their child's ongoing health status. One result was an increased reported level of stress by the mothers and other members of the family, including siblings, in the day-to-day management of the child with CHD. It is surprising and reassuring in the face of this ongoing concern that mothers were able to respond to their child in a way that produced positive parental and child outcomes. None of the children in the present study were in acute distress or hospitalized. The literature does suggest that parenting practices may be influenced by the stability of a child's chronic illness (Walker, Ford, & Donald, 1987). Also, the normalization advice these mothers consistently received from the clinic physicians and nurses, combined with the high level of social support they reported for their parenting, may have helped them cope more effectively with some of the negative aspects associated with their children's health conditions. Clearly, more research is needed regarding the impact of this heightened state of vigilance on the mother and other aspects of family functioning (e.g., marital satisfaction, maternal depression).

Limitations

There were a number of inherent limitations with this study that does limit its generalizability. The sample only included mothers and was largely from middle to upper middle socioeconomic class. The majority of the sample was Caucasian and included mothers who were well-educated. Other known determinants of parenting practices such as marital satisfaction, maternal mental health, and level of spousal support were not studied. The children were receiving excellent health care at a pediatric cardiology clinic in a large, urban children's hospital. Consequently, the present findings are most relevant to families with similar characteristics and who are receiving similar quality health care. The study measures, including the self-report instruments and the direct observations of the mother-child interactions, were carefully selected to be technically sound and meet the purposes of the study. However, all measures, particularly self-report measures, are limited by the number of areas they can assess; also, these measures may be susceptible to a socially desirable response set. For example, the child measures used sampled primarily behavioral and emotional development. Clearly other areas of child development such as adaptive, cognitive, language, and social development also are important but were not addressed in this study. Also, parents are unlikely to report or demonstrate on videotape child-rearing techniques that may violate social mores (e.g., yelling, spanking children). Finally, the issue of normalization surfaced as a potentially important variable in this study. However, despite this principle being well embraced by the pediatric cardiology clinic staff and routinely discussed with parents, we did not collect specific data on how much information parents received and the degree to which it influenced their child rearing philosophy or practices.

Implications for practice

There is no question that families meet a diagnosis of CHD with considerable anxiety and concern. However, with proper attention and support by an interdisciplinary health care team, the present study's results suggest that families can cope very well with this chronic childhood illness. Specific strategies that strengthen and maintain the parenting role should be included in nursing practice (Deatrick, Knafl, & Murphy-Moore, 1999). These include support, education and anticipatory guidance, and active listening.

Support

Social support is an important element in facilitating adaptation and adjustment to parenting a young child with CHD. The need for a comprehensive psychosocial and family assessment is indicated. This assessment should address social supports, strengths, and resources available to the family. Assisting parents to identify and develop formal and informal social support networks is a strategy that clinicians can use to help families. Family supports, church networks, and involvement with other community resources should be assessed. However, practitioners need to look beyond the "obvious" supports such as family and friends, and also consider support groups, relationships with health care providers, and on-line resources as other possible sources of support. Chat rooms, on-line support groups, and Internet access with other parents who have a child with a similar diagnosis may be helpful to some parents.

Education and anticipatory guidance

Parents need to understand the specific nature of their child's CHD, including the diagnosis, prognosis, treatment plan of care, and the health care strategies needed to use within the home. The complexity of the diagnosis and treatment compounds the need for education focused on the individual needs of the child and provided in the most meaningful way to the parents. This is built on an assessment of the parents' learning style and knowledge base. At the same time, parents need consistent encouragement to raise their children as "normal" as possible including age-appropriate expectations, nurturing, and discipline strategies. Discussing normalizing strategies and helping families identify and implement these behavioral strategies are clinical applications that can be implemented by the nurse. Normalization is a complex process and clinicians need a sound understanding of the attributes of normalization.

Active listening

The collection of the qualitative data in the present study was valuable and provided rich information regarding the parenting experience. Providing time for families to tell their stories is critical to understanding the lived experience of parenting a child with congenital heart disease. This need of mothers to tell stories and share their personal experience of parenting was also evident in the population of mothers of healthy children. An important role for the nurse is to help to slow the system down and to provide the time and opportunity for mothers to tell their stories. Through the listening of the stories, the nurse also is provided valuable information related to the stresses and strengths of the parenting experience. This can be helpful in designing strategies to support families during this life experience.

Further research

A final implication for nurses is the need to conduct further clinical research. The normalization process needs to be further studied as it affects individual families of children with chronic illnesses. The recent work of Knafl, Breitmayer, Gallo, and Zoeller (1996) is an example of such needed work. Further work also is needed on the heightened levels of maternal vigilance reported in this study and their short- and long-term impact on maternal health. An important related need is to identify interventions that may help mothers and fathers as they parent their young child with a chronic illness. In this time of diminished resources and cost containment, it is prudent to consider the value of nursing interventions as related to positive family outcomes. The role of the interdisciplinary team, but particularly the contributions of nurses in providing support, education, and care, cannot be discounted.

Acknowledgment

This research served as the basis for the first author's doctoral dissertation and was supported in part by a grant from the Children's Hospital Foundation, Milwaukee, WI.

References

Abidin, R.R. (1995). *Parenting Stress Index Manual* (3rd ed.). Charlottesville, VA: Pediatric Psychology Press.

Austin, J.K. (1991). Family adaptation to a child's chronic illness. *Annual Review of Nursing Research, 9*, 103-120.

Belsky, J. (1990). Parental and nonparental childcare and children's socioemotional development: A decade in review. *Journal of Marriage and the Family, 52*, 885-903.

Brenner, V., & Fox, R.A. (1999). An empirically derived classification of parenting practices. *The Journal of Genetic Psychology, 160*, 343-356.

Clawson, J.A. (1996). A child with a chronic illness and the process of family adaptation. *Journal of Pediatric Nursing, 11*, 52-61.

Collins, W.A., Maccoby, E.E., Steinberg, L., Hetherington, E.M., Bornstein, M.H. (2000). Contemporary research on parenting: The case for nature and nurture. *American Psychologist, 55*, 218-232.

Davis, C.C., Brown, R.T., Bakeman, R., & Campbell, R. (1998). Psychological adaptation and adjustment of mothers of children with congenital heart disease: Stress, coping, and family functioning. *Journal of Pediatric Psychology, 23*, 219-228.

Deatrick, J.A., Knafl, K.A., & Murphy-Moore, C. (1999). Clarifying the concept of normalization. *Image: Journal of Nursing Scholarship, 31*, 209-214.

Deatrick, J.A., Knafl, K.A., & Walsh, M. (1988). The process of parenting a child with a disability. *Image: Journal of Nursing Scholarship, 13*, 15-21.

DeMaso, D.R., Beardslee, W.R., Silbert, A.R., & Fyler, D.C. (1990). Psychological functioning in children with cyanotic heart defects. *Journal of Developmental Behavioral Pediatrics, 11*, 289-294.

DeMaso, D.R., Campis, L.K., Wypij, D., Bertram, S., Lipshitz, M., & Freed, M. (1991). The impact of maternal perceptions and medical severity on the adjustment of children with congenital heart disease. *Journal of Pediatric Psychology, 16*, 137-149.

Dolgin, M.J., Phipps, S., & Harow, E. (1990). Parental management of fear in chronically ill and healthy children. *Journal of Pediatric Psychology, 15*, 733-744.

Emery, J.L. (1989). Families with congenital heart disease. *Archives of Disease in Childhood, 64*, 150-154.

Eyberg, S.M., Bessmer, J.L., Newcomb, K., Edwards, D., & Robinson, E.A. (1994). *Dyadic parent-child interaction coding system–II: A manual* (4th rev.). Corte Madera, CA: Select Press.

Eyberg, S.M., & Ross, A.W. (1978). Assessment of child behavior problems: The validation of a new inventory. *Journal of Clinical Child Psychology, 7*, 113-116.

Fox, R.A. (1994). *Parent Behavior Checklist*. Austin, TX: ProEd. (Currently available from the author, Marquette University, School of Education, PO Box 1881, Milwaukee, WI 53201-1881; phone: 414-288-1469; email: robert.fox@marquette.edu.)

Fox, R.A., Platz, D.L., & Bentley, J.S. (1995). Maternal factors related to parenting practices, developmental expectations, and perceptions of child behavior problems. *The Journal of Genetic Psychology, 156*, 431-441.

Goldberg, S., Simmons, R.J., Newman, J., Campbell, K., & Fowler, R.S. (1991). Congenital heart disease, parental stress, and infant-mother relationships. *Journal of Pediatrics, 119*, 661-666.

Holaday, B. (1984). Challenges of rearing a chronically ill child. *Nursing Clinics of North America, 19*, 361-368.

Kazak, A.E. (1989). Families of chronically ill children: A systems and social-ecological model of adaptation and challenge. *Journal of Consulting and Clinical Psychology, 57*, 25-30.

Knafl, K., Breitmayer, B., Gallo, A., & Zoeller, L. (1996). Family response to childhood chronic illness: Description of management styles. *Journal of Pediatric Nursing, 11*, 315-326.

Krulik, T. (1980). Successful 'normalizing' tactics of parents of chronically ill children. *Journal of Advanced Nursing, 5*, 573-578.

Lobo, J.L. (1992). Parent-infant interaction during feeding when the infant has congenital heart disease. *Journal of Pediatric Nursing, 7*, 97-105.

Marino, B.L., & Lipshitz, M. (1991). Temperament in infants and toddlers with cardiac disease. *Pediatric Nursing, 17*, 445-448.

Maccoby, E.E. (1992). The role of parents in the socialization of children: An historical overview. *Developmental Psychology, 28*, 1006-1017.

Maccoby, E.E., & Martin, J.A. (1983). Socialization in the context of the family: Parent-child interaction. In P.H. Mussen (Ed.), *Handbook of Child Psychology* (pp. 1-101). New York: Wiley.

Moller, J.H., Neal, W.A., & Hoffman, W. (1988). *A Parent's Guide to Heart Disorders.* Minneapolis: University of Minnesota Press.

Newacheck, P.W., & Halfon, N. (1998). Prevalence and impact of disabling chronic conditions in childhood. *American Journal of Public Health, 88*, 610-617.

Newacheck, P.W., Stoddard, J.J., & McManus, M. (1993). Ethnocultural variations in the prevalence and impact of childhood chronic conditions. *Pediatrics, 91*, 1031-1039.

Nicholson, B., Anderson, M., Fox, R., & Brenner, V. (in press). One family at a time: A prevention program for at-risk parents. *Journal of Counseling and Development.*

O'Conner, T.G., Deater-Deckard, K., Fulker, D., Rutter, M. L., & Plomin, R. (1998). Genotype-environment correlations in late childhood and early adolescence: Antisocial behavioral problems and coercive parenting. *Developmental Psychology, 34*, 970-981.

Richman, N., & Graham, P.J., (1971). A behavioral screening questionnaire for use with three-year-old children. Preliminary findings. *Journal of Child Psychology and Psychiatry, 12*, 5-33.

Robinson, E.A., Eyberg, S.M., & Ross, A.W. (1980). The standardization of an inventory of child conduct problem behaviors. *Journal of Clinical Child Psychology, 9*, 22-28.

Sabbeth, B. (1984). Understanding the impact of chronic childhood illness on families. *Pediatric Clinics of North America, 31*, 47-56.

Simons, R.L., Beaman, J., Conger, R.D., & Chao, W. (1993). Childhood experience, conceptions of parenting, and attitudes of spouse as determinants of parental behavior. *Journal of Marriage and the Family, 55*, 91-106.

Svavarsdottir, E.K., & McCubbin, M. (1996). Parenthood transition for parents of an infant diagnosed with a congenital heart condition. *Journal of Pediatric Nursing, 11*, 207-216.

Steinberg, L., Lamborn, S., Darling, N., Mounts, N., & Dornbusch, S. (1994). Over-time changes in adjustment and competence among adolescents from authoritative, authoritarian, indulgent, and neglectful families. *Child Development, 65*, 754-770.

Tucker, M.A. & Fox, R.A. (1995). Assessment of families with mildly handicapped and nonhandicapped preschoolers. *Journal of School Psychology, 33*, 29-37.

Utens, E.M., Verhulst, F.C., Erdman, R.A., Meijboom, F.J., Duivenvoorden, H.J., Bos, E., Roelandt, J.R., & Hess, J. (1994). Psychosocial functioning of young adults after surgical correction for congenital heart disease in childhood: A follow-up study. *Journal of Psychosomatic Research, 38*, 745-758.

Van Dongen-Melman, J.E., & Sanders-Woudstra, J.A. (1986). Psychosocial aspects of childhood cancer: A review of the literature. *Journal of Child Psychology & Psychiatry & Allied Disciplines, 27*, 145-180.

Walker, L.S., Ford, M.B., & Donald, W.D. (1987). Cystic fibrosis and family stress: Effects of age and severity of illness. *Pediatrics, 79*, 239-246.

Publishing and Reprint Information

- *From Marquette University, Milwaukee, WI and the University of Southern Mississippi, Hattiesburg, MS.*

- *Address correspondence and reprint requests to Robert A. Fox, Professor, School of Education, Marquette University, PO Box 1881, Milwaukee, WI 53201-1881; E-mail: robert.fox@marquette.edu.*

- *0882-5963/02/1703-0004$35.00/0*

- *doi:10.1053/jpdn.2002.124111*

THE EFFECT OF TURNING AND BACKRUB ON MIXED VENOUS OXYGEN SATURATION IN CRITICALLY ILL PATIENTS

PATRICIA LEWIS, EVA NICHOLS, GLORIA MACKEY, ANECITA FADOL, LORINDA SLOANE, EVANGELINA VILLAGOMEZ, AND PATRICIA LIEHR

- *Objective: To examine the effect of a change in body position (right or left lateral) and timing of backrub (immediate or delayed) on mixed venous oxygen saturation in surgical ICU patients.*
- *Methods: A repeated-measures design was used to study 57 critically ill men. Mixed venous oxygen saturation was recorded at 1-minute intervals for 5 minutes in each of three periods: baseline, after turning, and after backrub. Subjects were randomly assigned to body position and timing of the backrub. Subjects in the immediate-backrub group were turned and given a 1-minute backrub. Mixed venous oxygen saturation was measured at 1-minute intervals for 5 minutes at two points: after the backrub and then with the patient lying on his side. For subjects in the delayed-backrub group, saturation was measured at 1-minute intervals for 5 minutes at two different points: after the subject was turned to his side and after the backrub.*
- *Results: Both position and timing of backrub had significant effects on mixed venous oxygen saturation across conditions over time. Subjects positioned on their left side had a significantly greater decrease in saturation when the backrub was started. At the end of the backrub, saturation was significantly lower in subjects lying on their left side than in subjects lying on their right side. The pattern of change differed according to the timing of the backrub, and return to baseline levels of saturation after intervention differed according to body position.*
- *Conclusions: Two consecutive interventions (change in body position and backrub) cause a greater decrease in mixed venous oxygen saturation than the two interventions separated by a 5-minute equilibrium period. Turning to the left side decreases oxygen saturation more than turning to the right side does. Oxygen saturation returns to clinically acceptable ranges within 5 minutes of an intervention. In patients with stable hemodynamic conditions, the standard practice of turning the patient and immediately giving a backrub is recommended. However, it is prudent to closely monitor individual patterns of mixed venous oxygen saturation, particularly in patients with unstable hemodynamic conditions.*

From Lewis, P., et al. (1997). The effect of turning and backrub on mixed venous oxygen saturation in critically ill patients. *American Journal of Critical Care, 6*(2), 132–140.

Backrubs and changes in body position are established interventions for enhancing patients' comfort, mobilizing pulmonary secretions, and improving tissue perfusion through pressure reduction.[1] Understanding the best strategies for combining these interventions may improve patients' outcomes and make the best use of nursing time.

BACKGROUND

Patients are commonly repositioned to the supine, right lateral, and left lateral positions before a backrub. The physiological effect of these interventions is questioned only if untoward changes are noted. Vital signs are routinely used to assess patients' responses to interventions such as changes in position and backrubs. Another useful measurement is mixed venous oxygen saturation (SvO_2), an indicator of oxygen delivery and consumption.

Normally, patients are given a backrub immediately after a change in body position. The consequences of multiple, sequential activities can be hemodynamic compromise. We were interested in comparing the effects on SvO_2 of turning with an immediate backrub and turning with a delayed backrub. The following research questions were addressed:

1. Does the change in SvO_2 after a 1-minute backrub in critically ill patients given the backrub immediately after turning differ from the change in SvO_2 in patients given the backrub 5 minutes after turning?
2. What is the effect of right and left lateral positions on SvO_2 in critically ill patients?

FRAMEWORK FOR THE STUDY

This study is based on the physiological principles underlying SvO_2. The SvO_2 indirectly reflects the balance between oxygen supply and tissue oxygen demands.[2–4] The normal range of SvO_2 is 60% to 80%. Determinants of SvO_2 are arterial oxygen saturation (SaO_2), hemoglobin levels, cardiac output, and tissue oxygen demands. Therefore, an uncompensated reduction in SaO_2, hemoglobin level, or cardiac output or increases in tissue oxygen consumption will result in a decreased SvO_2.[3]

The SaO_2 influences the SvO_2. Pathological pulmonary conditions that impair oxygen transfer at the alveolar-capillary membrane will result in less oxygen available for transport through the circulation. In addition, a deficit in hemoglobin reduces the oxygen-binding capacity of the blood and affects oxygen supply to the tissues. The cardiac output is the means for transporting oxyhemoglobin through the system. The fourth factor that influences SvO_2 is tissue oxygen demand. Tissue extraction of oxygen is increased in conditions such as fever, seizures, and shivering. Routine nursing care such as turning the patient, suctioning, weighing, bed baths, and backrubs may cause increased oxygen consumption. Rather than indicating a specific clinical event, SvO_2 reflects the balance between oxygen supply and demand. SvO_2 trends must be monitored closely to maximize medical and nursing intervention to optimize oxygenation and prevent an imbalance between oxygen supply and demand.[2–4]

LITERATURE REVIEW

Patients in the critical care environment are subject to conditions that may affect oxygen delivery and increase oxygen demand. Routine nursing interventions thought to be beneficial in preventing untoward outcomes may cause an imbalance between oxygen supply and demand. Investigators have studied the effects of a limited number of nursing activities on SvO_2 values. Body positioning has been the focus of much research[5–8] and has been a variable examined when other interventions such as bathing[9] and backrub[10] have been studied.

Shively[5] examined the effects of changes in body position and frequency of the changes on oxygenation in 30 subjects. Patients were randomly assigned to one of two groups. Patients in one group were turned every hour, whereas those in the other group were turned every 2 hours. All patients were turned in the following sequence: right lateral with the head of the bed elevated 20°, supine with the head of the bed at 45°, left lateral with the head of the bed at 20°, and supine with the head of the bed at 20°. SvO_2 values were recorded immediately after the turn (baseline values) and at 15 minutes, 1 hour, and 2 hours (second group only) after each change in position. The results showed no significant difference in SvO_2 between the two groups for time of turning ($P = .5757$) or for the four variations in body position ($P = .1351$). The difference in mean SvO_2 values measured at baseline and at 15 minutes after the turn was significant ($P = .0001$). There was also a significant difference between baseline values and the values determined 1 hour after changes in position ($P = .0001$). Interaction between position and time of measurement was significant (multivariate test: $F[6,23] = 6.87$, $P = .0003$; univariate test: $P = .0001$). Mean SvO_2 values were lowest immediately after a turn to the left lateral position.

Tidwell et al.[6] studied the effect of six position changes on 34 patients 4 to 8 hours after coronary artery bypass surgery. The initial change for all subjects was from supine to 30° head-of-bed elevation and back to supine. Thereafter, patients were randomized into two sequences: (1) right lateral, supine, left lateral, and then supine or (2) left lateral, supine, right lateral, and then supine. Subjects maintained each position for 30 minutes. SvO_2, SaO_2, and oxygen consumption were recorded simultaneously immediately before the position change, at each minute after the position change for 5 minutes, and at 15 and 25 minutes. Significant decreases in SvO_2 occurred with all changes from lateral and return to supine: supine to 45° right lateral recumbent ($P = .0$), 45° right lateral recumbent to supine ($P = .0002$), supine to 45° left lateral recumbent ($P = .0$), and 45° left lateral recumbent to supine ($P = .0031$). The greatest difference in mean SvO_2 values occurred in the interval between the time immediately before the change in position and the first minute after the change. Moving from supine to the right lateral recumbent position resulted in a decrease in mean SvO_2 of

6.1% whereas moving from supine to the left lateral recumbent position decreased SvO_2 by 5.6%.

Winslow et al.[7] studied the effect of change in body position in 174 patients as part of a multiinterventional study. All patients had pulmonary artery catheters in place. The subjects rested for 10 minutes and then were placed in the right or left side-lying position with the head of the bed at 20° and a pillow supporting them at a 60° angle from the bed. SvO_2 and heart rate were measured immediately after the turn and then at 1-minute intervals for 4 minutes. The decision to obtain the measurements with the subject in the right or left side-lying position was determined by the location of the tip of the subject's pulmonary artery catheter. Because the catheter tip was located in the right pulmonary artery in 85% of the subjects, only 15% of subjects were turned to the left side-lying position. Mean SvO_2 decreased from 67 ±8% at baseline to 61 ±10% ($P < .0001$) immediately after turning and gradually returned to 66 ±8% ($P < .002$) within 4 minutes. The decrease in SvO_2 immediately after turning was a change of 9% from baseline, which was more marked than the decrease in SvO_2 after other interventions. Analysis showed no significant difference in SvO_2 between subjects turned to the right and subjects turned to the left.

Copel and Stolarik[8] studied the effect of turning on 11 subjects after elective coronary artery bypass surgery. The majority of patients were turned from supine to the right lateral position and stayed in the lateral position for 6 to 16 minutes. SvO_2 decreased a mean of 11% immediately after the change in position. The difference in SvO_2 values obtained before and after turning was significant ($t = 9.87$, $df = 10$, $P < .01$) and persisted for a mean of 7.5 minutes.

Atkins et al.[9] studied the effect on SvO_2 of the timing of a bed bath in 30 subjects less than 24 hours after coronary artery bypass surgery. The study involved two bed baths consisting of a bathing phase and a turning phase early (mean, 3.6 hours) and late (mean, 18.5 hours) in the immediate postoperative period. Mean SvO_2 decreased from baseline values during the early and late bed baths by 1.6% and 1.9%, respectively. The mean SvO_2 during the turning phase decreased 9.2% and 12.1% from baseline, respectively. The return to baseline SvO_2 value after intervention required 3 to 4 minutes.

Tyler et al.[10] studied the effect of a 1-minute backrub on SvO_2 and heart rate in 173 critically ill patients as a part of the multiinterventional study[7] previously discussed. The backrub was the third intervention. All patients were placed supine, and baseline SvO_2 and heart rate were measured. The subjects were then turned to a lateral position. As previously described, the direction of the turn was determined by the location of the tip of the pulmonary artery catheter. The side-lying position was maintained for 15 minutes before the 1-minute backrub. Data were collected immediately after the backrub and then at 1-minute intervals for 4 minutes. After the backrub, mean SvO_2 decreased immediately from 67%, the baseline value, to 63% ($P = .0001$). SvO_2 returned to baseline within 4 minutes.

In summary, nursing interventions cause a significant decrease in SvO_2 immediately after the intervention is started. SvO_2 values usually return to baseline within 3 to 9 minutes, depending on the intervention.

METHODS

An experimental, repeated-measures, nested design was used. The study was approved by the institutional review board, and all subjects signed an informed consent document. Subjects were randomly assigned to right or left lateral position and then to an immediate or a delayed backrub. The sealed-envelope technique was used to assign position and then timing of backrub.

Sample and Setting

A convenience sample of 57 critically ill men in a surgical ICU at the Veterans Affairs Medical Center, Houston, Tex, was studied. No women were included in the sample because of the population of the study site. Power analysis[11] for repeated measures indicates that 23 subjects are needed to detect a medium effect at the .05 level of significance with a power of 0.80 and an estimated mean correlation among the repeated measures of 0.50 when only seven repeated measures are collected. This study had two grouping variables: position and immediacy of backrub. A minimum of 23 subjects was recruited into each group. This sample size provided more than adequate power, because 15 repeated measures were recorded for each subject.[11]

Subjects who had a fiber-optic pulmonary artery catheter in place, a baseline SvO_2 of 50% or higher, and an indwelling arterial catheter with normal waveform were eligible for inclusion in the study. Exclusion criteria included age less than 18 years, sepsis, pneumonectomy or lobectomy, mechanical assist devices in place, organ transplantation, and use of neuromuscular blocking agents. No subjects were excluded because of advanced age.

Instrumentation

Patients had fiber-optic thermodilution pulmonary artery catheters (the Explorer continuous venous oximeter, American Edwards Laboratories, Irvine, Calif) in place to measure SvO_2. Researchers have compared SvO_2 values obtained with fiber-optic thermodilution pulmonary artery catheters (in vivo) with values obtained in laboratory analyses (in vitro). For critically ill patients, correlations between in vivo and in vitro samples ranged from .89 to .97.[12–14] In addition to these high correlations, Baele et al.[12] found, in a sample of critically ill adults, that the catheters could be used for 102 hours with less than a 1% drift for every 24-hour period. Calibration of each catheter was completed within 24 hours before data collection.

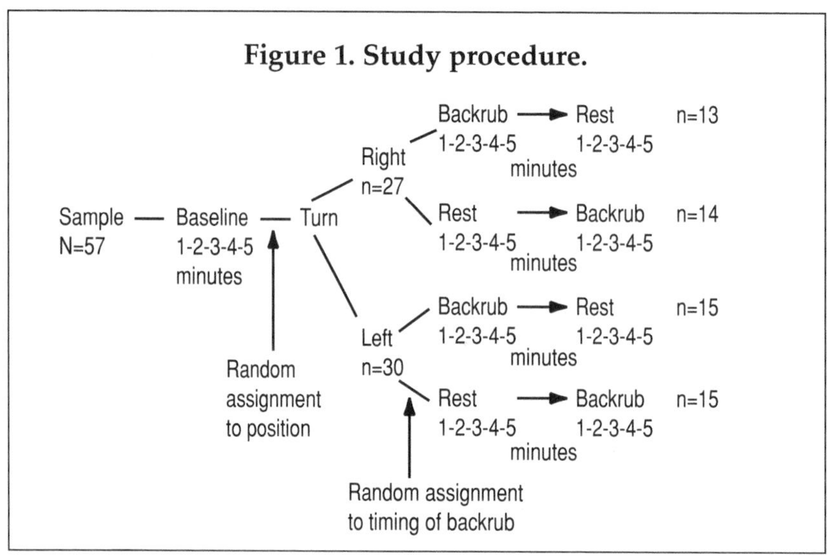

Procedure

After informed consent was obtained and randomization status decided, the patient was left undisturbed for 5 minutes lying supine with the head of the bed elevated 20° to 40°. Baseline SvO_2 was recorded at 1-minute intervals during this 5-minute period (Figure 1).

The patient was then turned to the left or right lateral position. A single data collector turned the patient and placed two folded standard pillows, one pillow behind the patient's back and one between the patient's knees. For patients in the delayed-backrub group, SvO_2 was again recorded at 1-minute intervals for 5 minutes after the change in body position. The patient was then given a 1-minute backrub. The backrub procedure was as follows:

1. The nurse poured lotion into his or her hands and warmed it by rubbing the hands together.
2. With lotion on both hands and palms flat and side by side, the nurse rubbed the patient's sacrum slowly in a circular motion for three circles.
3. The nurse then moved his or her hands slowly up the medial aspect of the patient's back and stopped at the scapular level.
4. Three circular motions were done in this region.
5. The nurse then moved his or her hands down the lateral aspect of the patient's back to massage the areas of the right and left iliac crests for three circular motions.

At the end of the backrub, one pillow was positioned behind the patient's back and one between the patient's knees, and SvO_2 was recorded from a digital readout at 1-minute intervals for 5 minutes.

Patients assigned to the immediate-backrub group were turned, and the backrub, as just described, was given immediately. After the backrub, SvO_2 was measured at 1-minute intervals for 5 minutes. There was then a 5-minute period during which 1-minute measurements were made while the patient remained in the lateral position.

Table 1. Means and standard deviations for factors affecting oxygen supply.

FACTOR	MEAN	SD
SaO_2 (%)	97.5	2.0
Hemoglobin (g/L)	89	12
Cardiac output (L/min)	6.6	1.2
Cardiac index (L/min per m^2)	3.23	0.58

Subjects

The mean age of the subjects was 60.9 years (standard deviation [SD] = 8.6; range, 40–79 years). Forty-nine subjects had had aortocoronary bypass surgery; 6, resection of an aortic aneurysm; 1, atrial septal repair; and 1, an esophogastrectomy. All subjects were in the surgical ICU at the time of the intervention. Forty-nine subjects were receiving oxygen by either face mask ($n = 22$) or nasal cannula ($n = 27$). Four subjects were receiving mechanical ventilation; 3 of these were receiving 5 cm of positive end-expiratory pressure. The remaining 4 subjects had no supplemental oxygen therapy. Mean SaO_2, hemoglobin level, cardiac output, and cardiac index are given in Table 1. Mean baseline heart rate for the sample was 98 beats per minute (SD = 15). There was no significant difference in the factors (SaO_2, hemoglobin level, or cardiac output) affecting oxygen supply or heart rate for the position group or the immediacy-of-backrub group. Table 2 lists the distribution of vasoactive therapies for the study subjects. Subjects receiving dopa-mine or IV nitroglycerin were equally distributed across groups (position or immediacy of backrub) as determined by chi-square analysis ($P > .05$). For all patients receiving dopamine, the dosage of the drug was a renal perfusion dosage and was not being titrated. Twenty-nine subjects were assigned to receive a delayed backrub; 28, an immediate backrub.

Table 2. Number of subjects receiving vasoactive therapy.

	NO. OF SUBJECTS	
MEDICATION	RECEIVING THERAPY	NOT RECEIVING THERAPY
Dopamine	39	18
Dobutamine	3	54
Norepinephrine	2	55
Epinephrine	1	56
Nitroprusside	1	56
Nitroglycerin	33	24

Data Analysis

Data were analyzed by using a 2 x 2 x 3 x 5 repeated-measures analysis of variance. The first two factors were grouping factors: (1) timing of backrub: immediate or delayed and (2) position: right or left. The second two factors were repeated measures

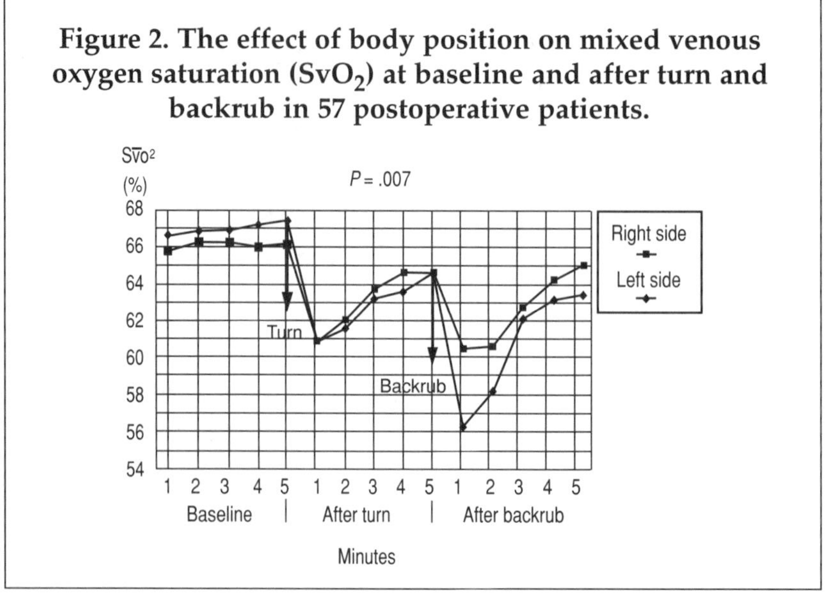

Figure 2. The effect of body position on mixed venous oxygen saturation (SvO_2) at baseline and after turn and backrub in 57 postoperative patients.

factors: (1) condition: baseline, back-rub, rest, and (2) time: 1 through 5 minutes. SvO_2 was the dependent measure. Greenhouse-Geisser adjusted degrees of freedom were used when appropriate. Scheffé tests ($P < .05$) were used to indicate significant differences between levels of SvO_2 at specific times during the protocol.

RESULTS

Both position ($F = 3.78$, $P = .007$) and immediacy of backrub ($F = 8.1$, $P = .000$) had significant effects on SvO_2 across conditions over time.

Except for the subjects who were on their left side for the backrub, when an intervention was introduced, (the turn itself or the beginning of the backrub), SvO_2 decreased significantly and then returned to baseline levels within 5 minutes as the condition persisted (Figure 2). Subjects positioned on their left side had a significantly greater (Scheffé tests, $P < .05$) decrease in SvO_2 when the backrub was initiated than subjects positioned on their right side (left side: mean = 64.6%, SD 6.7 to mean = 56.3%, SD 7.4; right side: mean 64.6%, SD = 8.9 to mean = 60.5%, SD = 11.2). At the end of the backrub, SvO_2 was significantly lower (Scheffé tests, $P < .05$) in subjects on their left side (mean = 63.4%, SD 7.2) than in subjects on their right side (mean = 65.0%, SD = 9.1). Further, for subjects on their left side, the final reading after the backrub was significantly lower than the final baseline value (Scheffé tests, $P < .05$). These lower SvO_2 values during the backrub occurred even though subjects lying on their left side had significantly higher (Scheffé tests, $P < .05$) values at baseline than subjects lying on their right side did.

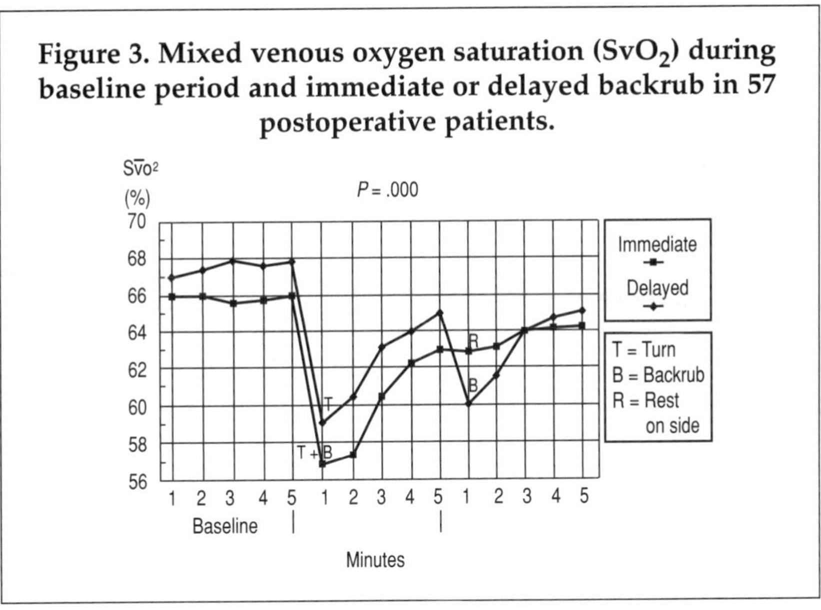

Figure 3. Mixed venous oxygen saturation (SvO_2) during baseline period and immediate or delayed backrub in 57 postoperative patients.

Subjects who had an immediate backrub had a significant decrease in SvO_2 (Scheffé tests, $P < .05$) when they were turned and the backrub was started (from mean = 65.9%, SD = 8.0 to mean = 56.7%, SD = 10.9). In this condition, the interventions (turn and backrub) occurred together. Steady increases in SvO_2 occurred during the backrub and continued into the control condition (Figure 3), during which the subject remained positioned on his side. In contrast, subjects who had a delayed backrub had significant decreases (Scheffé tests, $P < .05$) in SvO_2 both when turned (from mean = 67.7%, SD = 6.8 to mean = 58.8%, SD 7.6) and when the backrub was started (from mean 64.9%, SD 7.2 to mean 60.0%, SD = 7.7; Figure 3). SvO_2 increased during the 5 minutes after the introduction of each intervention. Therefore, the pattern of SvO_2 change was affected by the immediacy of the backrub.

DISCUSSION

Changes in Body Position

Although positioning to the right or left side is implicit in many nursing interventions, few studies have systematically studied the effect on SvO_2 of lying on the right or the left side. Shively[5] was the first to investigate this phenomenon. Two years after Shively's report, Tidwell et al.[6] reported another systematic investigation of the effect of positioning on oxygen delivery and utilization.

We systematically examined the effects of positioning on SvO_2 as a secondary research question. In the two previous investigations, all subjects were studied in both right and left lateral positions. In our study, subjects were randomly assigned to the right or the left lateral position. By itself, turning onto either side did not result in different SvO_2 values for the two groups (Figure 2). However, the combination of a turn to the left side plus a backrub produced the greatest decrease in SvO_2. The difference from the baseline SvO_2 was significant and persisted 5 minutes after the backrub.

The changes associated with positioning only are most like those reported by Tidwell et al.,[6] who found similar differences in SvO_2 when subjects were turned to the right or left side (6.1% decrease for turn to right and 5.6% decrease for turn to left). In our study, SvO_2 decreased 5.2% for a turn to the right and 6.4% for a turn to the left. Both our findings and those of Tidwell et al. contrast with the results of Shively,[5] who found that the lowest SvO_2 values occurred after a turn to the left side. Shively found a mean decrease of 7.7% (from 68.5% to 60.8%) in SvO_2 when subjects were positioned on their right side and a mean decrease of 11.1% (from 68.5% to 57.4%) when they were positioned on their left side. It is difficult to synthesize these different findings. At best, one can conclude that SvO_2 will decrease when a patient is turned, regardless of the side to which the patient is turned. In our study, 25 (44%) of the 57 subjects had SvO_2 values less than 60% associated with the turn. The lowest SvO_2 value was 47%, decreasing from a baseline of 52%. This subject's SvO_2 returned to 50% within 1 minute and was 52% at the end of the protocol. It is important to continue to assess individual SvO_2 values when patients are turned. The quick rebound of SvO_2 values noted in our study leads to questions about the clinical significance of the decrease in SvO_2 value to less than 60%. Even when mean values decreased into the 50% range, they did not remain that low for more than 3 minutes (Figure 2).

The most significant decreases in SvO_2 associated with turning occurred in subjects turned on their left side and given a backrub. This finding is difficult to explain on the basis of physiological parameters, because a backrub is a passive activity that demands no additional energy. Possibly, the left-sided position was associated with more pain. We did not collect data on the positioning of chest tubes, but evaluation of such data could add valuable information. If most chest tubes were positioned on the left side, the subtle added movements associated with a backrub might have exaggerated discomfort associated with positioning. Because the majority of patients were extubated at the time data were collected, it is expected that painful discomfort would have led to a request to be withdrawn from the study. No subjects asked to be withdrawn.

Although a significant difference persisted between baseline SvO_2 values (mean = 67.4%, SD = 7.4) and values obtained 5 minutes after the backrub (mean 63.4%, SD 7.2), this difference was not clinically important. Once again, although the mean values are within clinically acceptable limits, individual patterns of changes in SvO_2 should be closely assessed.

Immediacy of Backrub

In clinical practice, patients are turned, and backrubs are given. The most likely result of this sequence is that the patient actually gets a backrub. If the nurse leaves the patient and returns later for the backrub, intervening activities decrease the likelihood that a backrub will occur. Therefore, the question of when to give a backrub to facilitate optimal oxygen delivery and consumption and simultaneously conserve nursing time becomes important. In the delayed-backrub group, mean SvO_2 decreased from 64.9% to 60.0%. This change is not considered clinically significant, because the SvO_2 remained within the normal range. This reduction in SvO_2 may have been due to the combination of (1) the removal of the pillows, an intervention that includes a component of turning or repositioning; and (2) stimulation from the backrub. This result is similar to the findings in the study of Tyler et al.,[10] in which SvO_2 decreased significantly with the backrub even after a period of nonintervention. Interestingly, in our study, in 9 of the 25 subjects who had SvO_2 values less than 60% with the change in body position, initiation of the backrub increased the SvO_2 values. Four of the 9 had SvO_2 values greater than 60% with the start of the backrub. Three of these 4 were characterized by the recorder as very drowsy, very relaxed, or showing comfortable "moaning" during the backrub.

Two subjects had SvO_2 values that decreased to 33% with the backrub. Both subjects were in the immediate-backrub group. Their baseline SvO_2 values were 55% and 56%. One was positioned on his left side; the other, on the right side. The recorder stated that one of the patients was very tense (bearing down, grunting, holding breath). Both patients were extubated, alert, and receiving low-dose dopamine and nitroglycerin. The tense subject's SvO_2 returned to 53% in 4 minutes and to 56% after the additional 5 minutes in the side-lying position. The other subject's baseline SvO_2 was 52%. This subject's SvO_2 was 48% at 4 minutes after the turn to his right side and a backrub and 50% after the additional 5 minutes in the side-lying position. Cardiac output, cardiac index, and SaO_2 were within normal range for both subjects. The hemoglobin levels were 8.5 and 7.7 g/dL (85 and 77 g/L).

Six patients had an SvO_2 of 44% to 49% immediately after the backrub. Five of the six were in the immediate-backrub group. In two of the six, SvO_2 values were within normal limits by the end of the protocol. In the other four subjects, the SvO_2 values increased to 52% to 56% by the end of the protocol. The recorder stated that all four patients were tense, moaning, talking, coughing, or not comfortable. These behaviors may have increased oxygen consumption and limited the SvO_2 rebound seen in other subjects.

These examples show that multiple consecutive interventions may result in an even more significant decrease in SvO_2 for particular subjects. Atkins et al.[9] compared SvO_2 in patients having a continuous or an interrupted bed bath and concluded that consecutive interventions may have cumulative effects. For example, bathing the anterior surface of a patient's body is associated with minimal exertion by the patient, whereas turning the patient causes a significant decrease in SvO_2, and coughing, shivering, and agitation with activity such as turning can decrease the SvO_2 even more severely. Critically ill patients often require endotracheal suctioning, a procedure that can cause coughing or agitation. For comfort, patients may be turned to a lateral position after the suctioning and given a backrub. In this real-world example, patients are at risk for deterioration in their condition, especially if their baseline status was unstable. In our study, the mean SvO_2 decreased to 56.7% with the combined activity of a change in body position and a backrub. This decrease was not clinically significant. If the SvO_2 is 50% or less, oxygen delivery is marginal for oxygen demands, a situation that could cause deterioration in the patient's clinical condition, and possibly death.4 We do not mean that the SvO_2 should be less than 50%; rather, a momentary decrease in SvO_2 will be outweighed by the benefits of the intervention (e.g., suctioning, turning, backrub).

Our results do not support the approach of Tyler et al.[10] of waiting 15 minutes between turning the patient and given the backrub. Rather, we suggest that the standard practice of turning the patient and immediately giving a backrub be retained. The type of activity will determine the effect of multiple consecutive interventions on SvO_2. The less the exertion, the more likely it is that the patient will tolerate combined interventions. SvO_2 returned to baseline within 5 minutes of an intervention in most studies.[5–7,9,10,15] Copel and Stolarik[8] found that it took 7.5 minutes for subjects' SvO_2 to return to baseline values. In our study, SvO_2 immediately started to increase after an intervention but did not consistently return to baseline values within 5 minutes. The slower return occurred when subjects were on their left side. Although SvO_2 did not reach baseline values, mean SvO_2 did return to clinically acceptable levels within 5 minutes.

Generalizability of Findings

Several investigators[7,9,10] have studied factors that influence SvO_2, for example, SaO_2, hemoglobin level, cardiac output, and cardiac index. The reported values, like those of our study, were within normal limits. However, the mean hemoglobin level in subjects in our study was 89 g/L (SD = 12), whereas the mean in previous studies was 110 g/L. Our study was done in a time when blood products were given more judiciously than they had been in earlier times. Generally, the reported values of the factors that influence SvO_2 confirm the hemodynamic stability of the study populations, as do data on baseline SvO_2.

In all studies,[5–10] patients had mean baseline SvO_2 values within normal limits. In our study, the mean baseline SvO_2 was 66.0% to 67.8%. In only 8 (14%) of 57 subjects were baseline SvO_2 values less than 60%. The lowest baseline SvO_2 was 50%. Therefore our findings and those of other studies can be generalized only to a population of postoperative patients with hemodynamically stable conditions. During the past 5 years, SvO_2 monitoring has increasingly been used for patients with unstable hemodynamic conditions. The database that currently guides nursing intervention relative to oxygen delivery and consumption was developed with patients who had a stable hemodynamic status. The database should now be tested in patients with less stable conditions for whom SvO_2 monitoring is the current standard of care. The effects of these interventions most likely would be more dramatic in these compromised patients.

Implications for Practice

We recommend continuing the current practice of turning the patient and administering a backrub immediately in patients with hemodynamically stable conditions. Critical care nurses are more likely to provide this comfort measure when the intervention (backrub) occurs immediately after the turn, because this approach saves time; the nurse does not have to remember to return in 5 to 15 minutes to give the backrub. Furthermore, the patient is disturbed only once. Generally speaking, it does not matter whether the patient is turned to the right side or the left side. However, if the patient is turned to the left, monitoring throughout the next 10 minutes would be prudent to confirm that SvO_2 returns to baseline levels. Nurses should also assess the other factors that influence SvO_2, including SaO_2, cardiac output, and hemoglobin level. Despite the generalizations suggested by our results, we strongly recommend that nurses initially evaluate each patient's response to intervention.

In conclusion, nurses must be cognizant that each nursing intervention affects the physiological status of the patient. Furthermore, combined interventions such as turning and backrub may affect the patient's hemodynamic state more dramatically than individual interventions do. In this era of managed care, it is important to consider both the most effective and the most cost-efficient manner of delivering interventions. Our data indicate that for postoperative cardiac patients with hemodynamically stable conditions, the standard practice of turning the patients and immediately giving a backrub is the best use of nursing time and causes little disruption of oxygen delivery or consumption.

ACKNOWLEDGMENTS

We thank Cheryl Scarmardo, Andreas Siskind, and Kimberly Buckley for their time and expertise in preparing the manuscript, figures, and graphs.

References

1. Luckman J, Sorenson KC, eds. *Medical-Surgical Nursing: A Psychophysiologic Approach*. Philadelphia, Pa: WB Saunders Co; 1993.
2. Ahrens T, Rutherford K. *Essentials of Oxygenation*. Boston, Mass: Jones and Bartlett; 1993.
3. Cernaianu AC, Nelson LD. The significance of mixed venous oxygen saturation and technical aspects of continuous measurement. In: Edwards JD, Shoemaker WC, Vincent JL, eds. *Oxygen Transport: Principles and Practices.* Philadelphia, Pa: WB Saunders Co; 1993: 99–124.
4. White KM, Winslow EH, Clark AP, Tyler DO. The physiologic basis for continuous mixed venous oxygen saturation monitoring. *Heart Lung*. 1990; 19:548–551.
5. Shiveley M. Effect of position change on mixed venous oxygen saturation in coronary artery bypass surgery patients. *Heart Lung*. 1988; 17:51–59.
6. Tidwell, SL, Ryan WJ, Osguthorpe SG, Paull DL, Smith TL. Effect of position changes on mixed venous saturation in patients after coronary revascularization. *Heart Lung*. 1990: 19:574–578.
7. Winslow EH, Clark AP, White KM, Tyler DO. Effects of lateral turn on mixed venous oxygen saturation and heart rate in critically ill adults. *Heart Lung*. 1990; 19:557-566.
8. Copel LC, Stolarik A. Impact of nursing care activities on SvO_2 levels of postoperative cardiac surgery patients. *Cardiovasc Nurs*. 1991; 27:1–6.
9. Atkins PJ, Hapshe E, Riegel B. Effects of a bedbath on mixed venous oxygen saturation and heart rate in coronary artery bypass graft patients. *Am J Crit Care*. 1994; 3:107–115.
10. Tyler DO, Winslow EH, Clark AP, White KM. Effects of a 1-minute backrub on mixed venous oxygen saturation and heart rate in critically ill patients. *Heart Lung*. 1990; 19:562–565.
11. Barcikowski RS, Robey RR. Decisions in a single group repeated-measures analysis: statistical test and three computer packages. *Am Statistician*. 1984; 38:248–250.
12. Baele PL, McMichan JC, Marsh HM, Sill JC, Southorn PA. Continuous monitoring of mixed venous oxygen saturation in critically ill patients. *Anesth Analg*. 1982; 61:513–517.
13. Waller JL, Kaplan JA, Bauman DI, Craven JM. Clinical evaluation of a new fiberoptic catheter oximeter during cardiac surgery. *Anesth Analg*. 1982; 61:676–679.
14. Krouskop RW, Cabatu EE, Cheliah BP, McDonnell FE, Brown EG. Accuracy and clinical utility of an oxygen saturation catheter. *Crit Care Med*. 1983; 11:744–749.
15. Shinners PA, Pease MO. A stabilization period of 5 minutes is adequate when measuring pulmonary artery pressures after turning. *Am J Crit Care*. 1993; 2:474–477.

THE EFFECT OF A CORONARY ARTERY RISK EVALUATION PROGRAM ON SERUM LIPID VALUES AND CARDIOVASCULAR RISK LEVELS

SANDRA L. BRUCE AND SUSAN K. GROVE

In this study, serum lipid and cardiovascular risk levels of 195 military men and women were measured immediately before and 6 months after participation in a coronary artery risk evaluation (C.A.R.E.) program. Mean total cholesterol levels decreased from 257 mg/dl to 223 mg/dl ($t_{(194)} = -16.76$, $p = 0.00$), low-density lipoprotein levels decreased from 170 mg/dl to 141 mg/dl ($t_{(194)} = -15.22$, $p = 0.00$), and high-density lipoprotein levels increased from 45 mg/dl to 48 mg/dl ($t_{(194)} = 3.27$, $p = 0.01$). Cardiovascular risk categories (based on serum lipid levels) were lowered from high to moderate risk in 54 subjects, high to low risk in 19 subjects, and moderate to low risk in 31 subjects ($\chi^2 = 98.28$, $p = 0.00$). This study demonstrates that health education programs such as the C.A.R.E. Program can have a significant impact on serum lipid levels and cardiovascular risk levels and can potentially improve the health of high-risk populations.

Cardiovascular diseases cause nearly one of every two deaths in adults 45 years and older (American Heart Association, 1988). "It ranks first in terms of social security disability and second only to all forms of arthritis for limitation of activity, and to all forms of cancer combined for total hospital stays. In direct health care costs, lost wages, and productivity, coronary artery disease (CAD) costs the United States more than $60 billion a year" (Lipid Research Clinics [LRC] Program, p. 351).

Risk factors for CAD include male gender, family history of premature CAD, diabetes mellitus, hypertension, high cholesterol, cigarette smoking, and obesity (Expert Panel, 1988). The first three risk factors cannot be changed; however, the last four factors can be modified. Education can promote changes in daily living that reduce the risk for CAD (Glanz, 1988). The National Center for Health Statistics reports that slightly over 50% of Americans aged 20 to 74 have total blood cholesterol levels above the desirable level of 200 mg/dl. About 25% of the adult population is at high risk of CAD owing to levels of 240 mg/dl or greater and are candidates for intervention (Sempos, Fulwood, Hianes, & Cleeman, 1989).

Cholesterol is transported in the blood by lipoproteins. The low-density lipoprotein (LDL) carries most of the blood's cholesterol; high levels of LDL lead to atherosclerosis. The high-density lipoprotein (HDL) carries less of the blood cholesterol and helps prevent cholesterol deposition in the arteries (Kwiterovich, 1989). The goal of all risk-factor reduction strategies is to change blood lipid profiles from a "bad" one (high

From Bruce, S.L., & Grove, S.K. (1994). The effect of a coronary artery risk evaluation program on serum lipid values and cardiovascular risk levels. *Applied Nursing Research, 7*(2), 67–74.

LDL, low HDL) to a "good" one (low LDL, high HDL). The purpose of this descriptive study was to compare a military population's mean levels of total serum cholesterol, LDL, HDL, and risk for cardiovascular disease (based on serum lipid levels) before and 6 months after a coronary artery risk evaluation (C.A.R.E.) program.

BACKGROUND

The Framingham study provided the first strong link between cholesterol, lipoproteins, and coronary artery disease in men and women (Kannel, Castelli, Gordon, & McNamara, 1971). Study results suggested that total serum cholesterol was the best indicator of CAD; people with elevated LDL cholesterol were more at risk than those with low levels of LDL. In addition, people with normal total cholesterol and low HDL cholesterol were more prone to cardiovascular disease than those with normal cholesterol and high HDL. For people at high risk for CAD, drugs were used to reduce their risk levels.

The LRC Coronary Primary Prevention Trial (1984) was a double-blind study that examined the effect of the lipid-lowering drug cholestyramine on the serum lipid levels and incidence of coronary events (number of heart attacks and deaths due to CAD) in approximately 4,000 men. Both the treatment group and the control group were placed on a low-saturated fat diet. Results from this trial demonstrated an 8.5% reduction in LDL cholesterol for the treatment group; this reduction was associated with a 19% reduction in CAD risk (LRC, 1984). These findings suggested that for every 1% reduction in blood cholesterol, CAD risk is reduced by 2% (National Institutes of Health [NIH], 1985).

The results of three clinical trials, the LRC Coronary Primary Prevention Trial (1984), The National Heart, Lung, and Blood Institute's Coronary Trial (NIH, 1985), and the Cholesterol-Lowering Atherosclerosis Study (Blankenhorn et al., 1987) found that an increase in HDL cholesterol produced a reduction in coronary artery disease in addition to the beneficial effect of lowering the LDL level (Kwiterovich, 1989). The Helsinki Heart Study was a rigorous experimental study on 4,081 asymptomatic, hypercholesterolemic men treated with a cholesterol-lowering diet or diet plus gemfibrozil (Fricke et al., 1987). Results demonstrated an 8% increase of HDL cholesterol and a 34% decrease in incidence of coronary events in the latter group. These results suggest that for every 1% increase in HDL level, there is about a 3% decrease in risk for CAD. This does not negate the additive effect of all risk factors in the development of CAD, but rather highlights the influence that serum LDL and HDL have in predicting risk (Cornett & Watson, 1984).

Nonpharmacological interventions also may be effective in reducing serum cholesterol. Peterson, Lefebvre, and Ferreira (1986) reported a 10.9% cholesterol reduction 6 months after intervention (one-time screening, counseling, health referrals, and follow-up screening), and Quigley (1986) reported a 14% reduction in total cholesterol 8 months after intervention (screening, two 1-hour education sessions about cholesterol, and rescreening). The New York Telephone Company Trial reported a greater decrease in cholesterol (8.8%) in the treatment group (8-week education program that included nutrition education and training in self-management skills) than the control group (2.4%), as well as significantly greater weight loss (Bruno, Arnold, Jacobson, Winick, & Wynder, 1983). Each of these studies demonstrated positive effects from risk reduction education (Glanz, 1988).

Blair, Bryant, and Bocuzzi (1988) reported findings from an 18-month study conducted in a nurse-managed clinic for hyperlipidemic military personnel and their dependents. The subjects ($N = 86$) had cardiovascular disease and were treated with a cholesterol lowering diet and drugs. Thirty-two (37%) of the subjects were able to lower their mean cholesterol from 299 mg/dl to 241 mg/dl (19% reduction) on dietary therapy alone, and 54 (63%) achieved a 25% decrease in mean cholesterol from 310 mg/dl to 231 mg/dl on diet and drug therapy. This study highlighted the effectiveness of nursing interventions in individuals with hyperlipidemia.

In March 1988, the Strategic Air Command Surgeon General directed medical facilities to provide a means for military members to voluntarily obtain information regarding their lipid status and risk for cardiovascular disease. The staff of an outpatient primary care clinic in Texas developed the C.A.R.E. program to effect positive health outcomes (reduction in CAD risk) through a lipid screening and education intervention. This study evaluated the relationship between an education intervention (the C.A.R.E. program) and health outcomes (decreased serum lipids and cardiovascular risk). The following research question was developed for the study: What is the difference in the mean total serum cholesterol, LDL cholesterol, and HDL cholesterol and cardiovascular risk levels of military members before and after participation in the C.A.R.E. program?

METHOD

Sample: The setting was the outpatient primary care clinic of a 140-bed military hospital that serves men and women who are active duty or retired from active duty as well as their dependents over the age of 16 years. The C.A.R.E. program was advertised in the clinic lobby and the base newspaper as a service for anyone interested in learning about their lipid levels and risk of heart disease. Although it was mandated by the Strategic Air Command Surgeon General to provide this service, participation was voluntary.

The Expert Panel of the National Heart, Lung, and Blood Institute's National Cholesterol Education Program (NCEP) has established guidelines for detecting, evaluating, and treating hypercholesterolemia. These guidelines formed the standards for the intervention used in this study (Figure 1). As a result of the growing understanding about the role of cholesterol in CAD, the NCEP was developed to inform health professionals and the public about the importance of monitoring serum cholesterol levels (Expert Panel, 1988).

The C.A.R.E. program was conducted for a period of one year, and a total of 483 individuals were voluntarily screened. Fifteen of these individuals were referred immediately to the internal medicine clinic because of dangerously high lipid values

Figure 1. C.A.R.E. guidelines adapted from the NCEP. (Reprinted from Expert Panel, 1988.)

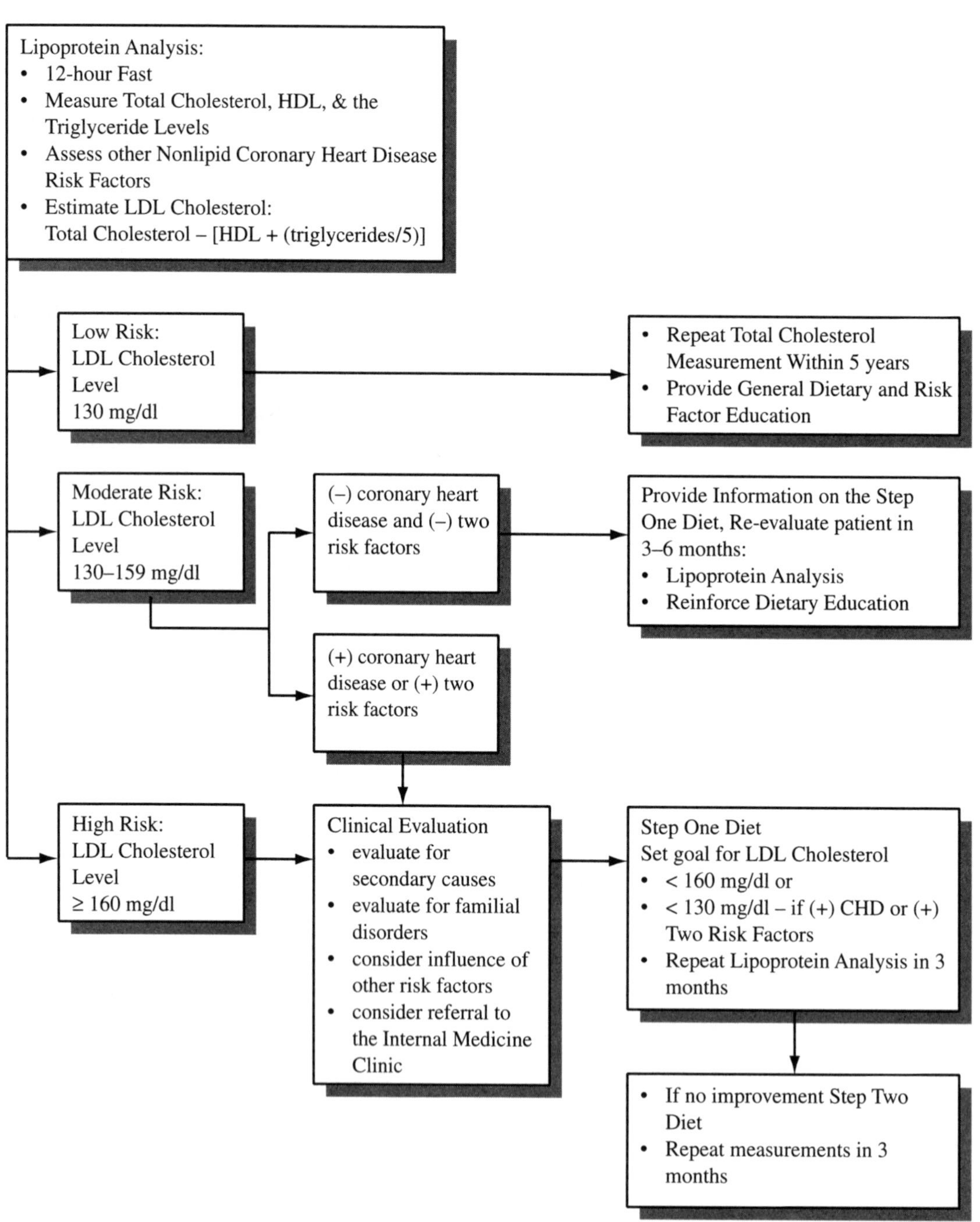

(serum cholesterol greater than 300 mg/dl) and two or more nonlipid risk factors. These individuals were not included in the study sample. Those with cholesterol values less than 200 mg/dl (and the absence of other nonlipid risk factors) were considered low risk. Owing to their low risk, these individuals (n = 122) were instructed to have follow-up blood levels drawn in one year and were not included in the sample. One hundred twenty-seven individuals did not return for follow-up evaluation and were not included in the study sample. Twenty-four of the individuals screened did not meet the following sample criteria: (a) greater than 16 years of age; (b) military members (active duty, retired, or dependent); (c) not under pharmacological treatment for hyperlipidemia; (d) English-speaking; (e) triglycerides under 400 mg/dl (this criterion was set because the calculation for LDL is not accurate for individuals for triglyceride values greater than 400 mg/dl); (f) nondiabetic; and (g) no current referrals to other health providers. Of the 483 individuals screened, 195 became research subjects. A power analysis was performed to confirm the adequacy of the sample size (Cohen, 1988).

The sample consisted of 92 men and 103 women and included 36 married couples. The subjects ranged from 20 to 80 years of age, with a mean age of 53.33 years (± 13 SD). Information about the subjects' body mass index (BMI), systolic blood pressure (SBP), diastolic blood pressure (DBP), heart rate, and glucose are provided in Table 1. The means for these variables were within normal limits.

Procedure: The data (serum lipid values and individual risk factor information) were obtained through retrospective medical record review and coded in order to protect the subject's identity. Measurements of the total serum cholesterol, the HDL, the LDL, and the estimated cardiovascular risk level were compared before and 6 months after participation in the program. The C.A.R.E. program was a voluntary program that offered screening, evaluation, and cardiac risk reduction education to all eligible military personnel. Screening consisted of an interview by the nurse manager of the program to determine individual risk factors and to provide instructions for obtaining a

Table 1. Means, standard deviations, and ranges of the physiological attributes of the sample (92 men and 103 women).

Attribute	$\bar{X}$	**SD**	**Range**
[a]BMI (Kg/cm^2)	25.03	2.82	19.57–37.19
SBP (mmHg)	135.08	17.72	100–178
DBP (mmHg)	82.98	8.51	54–102
Heart Rate	85.33	8.11	64–104
Serum Glucose (mg/dl)	97.83	13.83	72–130

Abbreviations: SBP, systolic blood pressure; DBP, diastolic blood pressure; BMI, body mass index, [a]BMI: 19 = lean; 25 = average; 31 = heavy (Kwiterovich, 1989).

fasting lipid profile and glucose. The participants also had their height, weight, and blood pressure checked. Each person then was enrolled in the next available C.A.R.E. class.

In the evaluation phase, the program nurse, in conjunction with the clinic physician, assessed the person's cardiac risk status based on reported risk factors and the results of the serum lipid profile, according to NCEP guidelines. Each C.A.R.E. participant was determined to have low, moderate, or high risk for cardiovascular disease. Recommendations were made based on this risk classification and individual considerations. These recommendations included dietary guidelines, exercise guidelines, follow-up instructions, and in some cases, formal referrals to other resources.

The educational phase of the program involved attending a C.A.R.E. class. This 90-minute class provided instruction concerning cardiovascular health, emphasizing the relationship between daily living behaviors, and identification of risk factors that determine one's risk for heart disease. At the beginning of this group session, each participant was given a handout that included the following information: their serum lipid profile results; their risk classification (high, moderate, or low); and specific individualized recommendations. The results of the lipid profiles and risk-level evaluations were explained in detail. Dietary instruction on the Step-One Diet (Table 2) was provided, as recommended by the Expert Panel (1988). Copies of the Step-One Diet were given to each person. General behavioral changes were recommended to the participants, such as reducing sedentary behaviors and maintaining ideal body weight. At the close of the class, recommendations and follow-up instructions were discussed with each participant individually. The subjects also received follow-up screening and counseling (based on rescreening results) 6 months after the start of the program.

Table 2. Dietary guidelines to lower blood cholesterol.

	Recommended Intake	
Nutrient	**Step-One Diet**	**Step-Two Diet**
Total Fat	<30% of total calories	<30% of total calories
Saturated fatty acids	<10% of total calories	<7% of total calories
Polyunsaturated fatty acids	0% to 10% of total calories	0% to 10% of total calories
Carbohydrates	10% to 15% of total calories	10% to 15% of total calories
Protein	50% to 60% of total calories	50% to 60% of total calories
Cholesterol	10% to 20% of total calories	10% to 20% of total calories
	<300 mg/day	<200 mg/day
	To achieve and maintain desirable weight	To achieve and maintain desirable weight

Reprinted from Expert Panel (1998).

Measures: A standardized protocol for lipid data collection, prescribed by the NCEP, was followed by each subject: (a) fast for 12 hours; (b) maintain stable dietary patterns for at least three weeks; (c) maintain stable body weight; (d) be neither ill nor pregnant; and (e) have no recent history of myocardial infarction, less than 3 months. The laboratory values of total serum, LDL, and HDL cholesterol from this agency met the referenced criteria (± 3% of the true value) set by the NCEP. The true value is an accepted reference value, established by the National Bureau of Standards (NBS) or the Centers for Disease Control (Finney, 1990). The level of LDL cholesterol was calculated using the following equation developed by Friedewald, Levy, and Fredrickson (1972): Total cholesterol – [HDL cholesterol + (triglycerides/5)] = LDL.

RESULTS

The most prevalent nonlipid risk factor present for this sample was a family history of coronary artery disease; 73 (37.4%) of the subjects reported that definite myocardial infarction or sudden death had occurred before the age of 65 years in a parent or sibling. Incidence of other reported risk factors were as follows: cigarette smoking, 22.1%; hypertension (SBP 140 mmHg; DBP 90 mmHg), 15.9%; obesity (greater than or equal to 30% over ideal body weight), 5.6%; and diagnosed coronary artery disease, 3.1%.

Six months after participation in the C.A.R.E. program, the mean total cholesterol was reduced by 33.82 mg/dl ($t(194) = -16.76$, $p = 0.00$), and the mean LDL level was reduced by 28.97 mg/dl ($t(194) = -15.22$, $p = 0.00$). The mean HDL cholesterol was increased by 2.75 mg/dl ($t(194) = 3.27$, $p = 0.001$) (Table 3).

Table 3. Baseline and follow-up mean cholesterol levels (mg/dl) in study population (92 men and 103 women).

	Baseline		Follow-Up			
Type of Cholesterol	$\bar{x}$	**SD**	$\bar{x}$	**SD**	**t VALUE**	**p**
Total serum cholesterol	257.20	36.43	223.38	34.05	–16.75	0.0000
LDL cholesterol	170.40	36.52	141.43	32.24	–15.22	0.0000
HDL cholesterol	44.83	15.01	47.58	13.00	+3.27	0.0012

Abbreviations: LDL, low-density lipoprotein; HDL, high-density lipoprotein.

Figure 2. Percentage of subjects in each cardiovascular risk category before and after treatment (*P* = .0000).

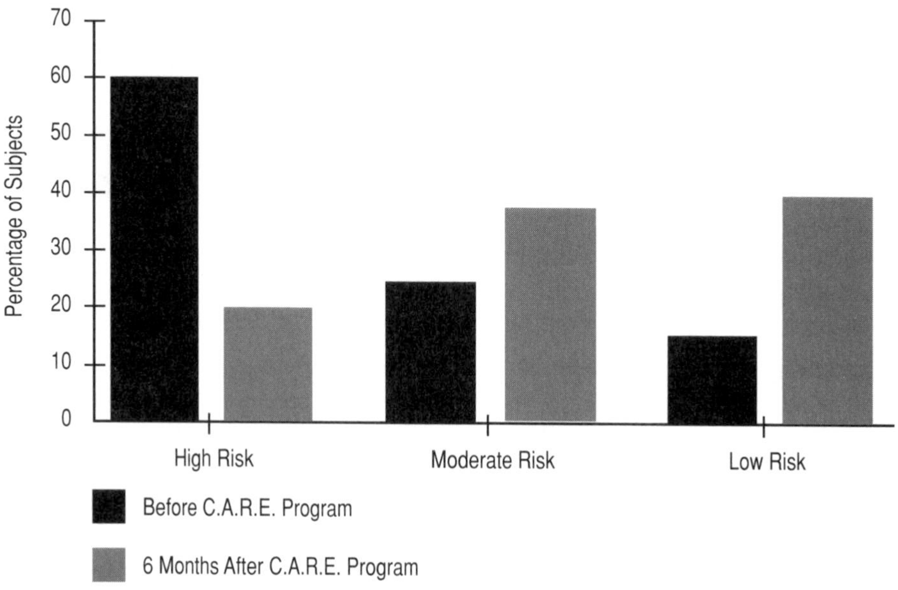

The risk levels of the subjects before and 6 months after the C.A.R.E. program were compared. Using a 3 x 3 – chi-square table, the sample was categorized into low, moderate, and high risk for cardiovascular disease based on the serum lipid profile and nonlipid risk factors before and after participation (Figure 2). The number of subjects in the high-risk category before participation was 116 (59.5%) and was reduced to 45 (23.1%) after participation; 50 (25.6%) were in the moderate-risk category before participation and 71 (36.4%) after participation; and 29 (14.9%) were in the low-risk category before participation and 79 (40.5%) after participation. The increased number of subjects in the moderate-risk group after participation is accounted for by the movement of high-risk individuals to the moderate-risk category. Cardiovascular risk categories were lowered from high to moderate risk in 54 subjects; high to low risk in 19 subjects; and moderate to low risk in 31 subjects; 43 remained high risk; 17 remained moderate risk; and 29 remained in low risk. Only two individuals went from moderate to high risk. Significant changes in risk factor categorization were noted using an extension of the McNemar Test for Significance of Changes (Bowker, 1948; McNemar, 1947). The value obtained (χ^2 greater than 98.285, $p = 0.00$) was 12.6 times larger than the critical value of $\chi^2 = 7.815$ (0.95, $df = 3$), demonstrating a significant difference in the cardiovascular risk levels of the group posttreatment.

DISCUSSION

The screening process was beneficial in identifying individuals with health risks. Fifteen individuals were referred for medical intervention because of dangerously high cardiovascular risk levels. Eleven other subjects were referred for evaluation of hypertension, and 6 subjects were referred for elevated fasting serum glucose levels.

As expected, strong correlations were found between cardiovascular risk and the total cholesterol level ($r = .67$, $p = .000$; 44% variance explained) and the LDL cholesterol level ($r = .80$, $p = .000$; 64% variance explained). However, HDL cholesterol did not correlate significantly with cardiovascular risk level ($r = -.12$; 1.5% of the variance explained), which is unexpected because the literature supports this correlation (Lipid Research Clinics Program, 1984; Fricke et al., 1987; Levy et al., 1984; Pocock, Shaper, & Phillips, 1989).

A significant 13% decrease in the mean total serum cholesterol level occurred after participation in the C.A.R.E. program. Based on the premise that a 1% reduction in serum cholesterol produces a 2% reduction in cardiovascular risk, the participants in this study could have achieved an overall 26% reduction in risk for coronary heart disease (LRC, 1984; NIH, 1985). Several nonpharmacological cardiovascular education intervention studies reported similar reductions in total serum cholesterol levels. Peterson and colleagues (1986) reported a 11% mean reduction of total cholesterol 6 months after interventions; Quigley (1986) reported a 14% reduction in total cholesterol levels 8 months after an education program; and Bruno and colleagues (1983) reported a 9% reduction 6 months after intervention. Thus, the 13% reduction in total serum cholesterol after the C.A.R.E. program was consistent with other nonpharmacological education interventions.

Mean LDL levels decreased 17% after participation in the C.A.R.E. program. An LDL level greater than 160 mg/dl constitutes high risk for cardiovascular disease regardless of the presence of other risk factors. The participants in the C.A.R.E. program reduced their mean LDL level from 170.40 to 140.43 mg/dl (17% reduction) and on the basis of this factor alone lowered their overall risk classification from high to moderate.

Mean HDL cholesterol level increased 5.8% after participation in the C.A.R.E. program. Results from the Helsinki Heart Study suggest that for every 1% increase in HDL level, a 3% decrease in risk for CAD occurs (Fricke et al., 1987). According to this premise, the study subjects decreased their risk for coronary heart disease by 17.4%.

The majority (99.5%) of the subjects either decreased their cardiovascular risk classification or remained in the same classification after participation in the C.A.R.E. program. Only 2 (1%) of the 195 participants increased their risk levels (from moderate to high risk). This could be attributed to noncompliance to the C.A.R.E. program guidelines or familial hyperlipidemia (Kwiterovich, 1989). The latter may require pharmacological intervention. Overall, positive changes in the participants' blood lipid levels and cardiovascular risk classification were noted after participation in the C.A.R.E. program.

Several factors must be considered when interpreting these findings. In this descriptive study, the original risk was based on the serum lipid profile and the presence of nonlipid risk factors as indicated by the Expert Panel (1988), and the changes in risk classification are based on changes in the lipid values only. Other variables known to affect cardiovascular risk (e.g., exercise, smoking, hypertension, body weight) were not reexamined after participation in the C.A.R.E. program. There may have been an even greater magnitude of change in risk classification if other risk factors were measured postparticipation. "Regression toward the mean" may have been responsible for some of the cholesterol reduction because single determinations were used to establish baseline and end-of-participation blood lipid levels (Green & Lewis, 1986). The findings may demonstrate an association between the C.A.R.E. program and the improvements in serum lipid values for the sample. However, quasi-experimental studies with control groups are needed to examine the full impact of the program.

Because the study was limited to 6 months after participation in the C.A.R.E. program, long-term trends were not examined. Future research should include longitudinal studies to assess the degree to which behavior changes are sustained over time. Examining different populations such as minorities, women, children, and the elderly would strengthen the findings. Finally, a cost-benefit analysis could highlight potential savings in terms of health-care costs for high-risk individuals.

Health education has long been an integral component of professional nursing. Indeed, nurses can be viewed as a primary source of health information. Education does not have to be lengthy to be beneficial. The simple changes corresponding to those of the NCEP's Step-One Diet can be recommended by a nurse in a few minutes. The results do support the use of educational programs in addition to risk factor assessment in reducing cardiac risk levels. Education can be effective in improving lipid profiles and potentially decrease the incidence of CAD. Decreasing risk for CAD and the associated loss of productivity, disability, and death could enhance quality of life. This study demonstrates that nurse-managed health education programs such as the C.A.R.E. program can have dramatic impact on individuals' health and can potentially improve quality of life for high-risk populations.

From the Sheppard Air Force Base, and the University of Texas at Arlington, TX.

Sandra L. Bruce, MSN, RN, CCRN: Major, United States Air Force, Nurse Corps. Sheppard Air Force Base, TX; Susan K. Grove, PhD, RN: Professor, Assistant Dean, The University of Texas at Arlington School of Nursing.

Address reprint requests to Sandra L. Bruce, MSN, RN, CCRN, Major, United States Air Force, 383d Medical Training Squadron/NTOE, 939 Missile Rd., Suite 3, Sheppard Air Force Base, TX, 76311-2262.

0897-1897/94/0702-0004$0.00/0

References

American Heart Association (1988). *Recommendations for treatment of hyperlipidemia in adults*. Dallas, TX: American Heart Association.

Blair, T.P., Bryant, J., & Bocuzzi, S. (1988). Treatment of hypercholesterolemia by a clinical nurse using a stepped-care protocol in a nonvolunteer population. *Archives of Internal Medicine, 148*, 1046–1048.

Blankenhorn, D.H., Nessim, S.A., Johnson, R.L., San Marco, M.E., Azen, A.P., & Cashen-Hemphill, L. (1987). Beneficial effects of combined colestipol-niacin therapy on coronary atherosclerosis and coronary artery vs bypass grafts. *JAMA, 257*, 3233–3240.

Bowker, A.H. (1948). A test for symmetry in contingency tables. *Journal of the American Statistical Association*, 43, 572–574.

Bruno, R., Arnold, C., Jacobson, L., Winick, M., & Wynder, E. (1983). Randomized trial of a nonpharmacologic cholesterol reduction program at the worksite. *Preventive Medicine, 12*, 523–532.

Cohen, J. (1988). *Statistical power analysis for the behavioral sciences* (2nd ed.). Hillsdale, NJ: Lawrence and Earlbam Associates.

Expert Panel (1988). *Report of the National Cholesterol Education Program Expert Panel on detection, evaluation, and treatment of high blood cholesterol in adults* (US Dept of Health and Human Resources Publication No. NIH 88-2925.) Washington, DC: National Heart, Lung, and Blood Institute.

Finney, C.P. (1990). Measurement issues in cholesterol screening: An overview for nurses. *Journal of Cardiovascular Nursing*, 5(2), 10–22.

Friedewald, W.T., Levy, R.I., & Fredrickson, D.S. (1972). Estimation of the concentration of low-density lipoprotein cholesterol in plasma, without the use of the preparative ultracentrifuge. *Clinical Chemistry*, 18, 499–502.

Fricke, M.H., Elo, O., Haapa, K., Heinonen, O.P., Heinsalmi, P., Helo, P., Huttunen, J.K., Kaitaniemi, P., Koskinen, P., Manninen, V., Maenpaa, H., Malkonen, M., Manttari, M., Novola, S., Paternick, A., Pikkarainen, J., Romo, M., Sjoblom, T., & Nikkila, E.A. (1987). Helsinki heart study: Primary prevention trial with gemfibrozil in middle-aged men with dyslipidemia. *New England Journal of Medicine, 317*, 1237–1245.

Glanz, K. (1988). Patient and public education for cholesterol reduction: A review of strategies and issues. *Patient Education and Counseling, 12*, 235–257.

Green, L.W., Kreuter, M.W., Deeds, S.G., & Partridge, K.B. (1980). *Health education and planning: A diagnostic approach*. Palo Alto, CA: Mayfield.

Green, L.W., & Lewis, F.M. (1986). *Measurement and evaluation in health education and promotion*. Palo Alto, CA: Mayfield.

Kannel, W.B., Castelli, W.P., Gordon, T., & McNamara, P.M. (1971). Serum cholesterol, lipoproteins, and the risk of coronary heart disease: The Framingham study. *Annals of Internal Medicine, 74*, 1–12.

Kwiterovich, P. (1989). *Beyond cholesterol: The Johns Hopkins complete guide for avoiding heart disease.* Baltimore, MD: Johns Hopkins University Press.

Levy, R.F., Brensike, J.F., Epstein, S.E., Kelsey, S.F., Passamani, E.R., Richardson, J.W., Loh, I.K., Stone, N.I., Aldrich, R.F., Battaglini, J.W., Moriarty, D.J., Fisher, M.L., Friedman, L., Friedewald, W., & Detre, K.M. (1984). The influence of changes in lipid values induced by cholestyramine and diet on progression of coronary artery disease results of the NHLBI, type II coronary intervention study. *Circulation, 69,* 325–327.

Lipid Research Clinics Program (1984). The lipid research clinics coronary primary prevention trial results I. Reduction in incidence of coronary heart disease to cholesterol lowering. *JAMA, 251,* 351–364.

McNemar, Q. (1947). Note on the sampling error of the difference between correlated proportions of percentages. *Psychometrika, 12,* 153–157.

National Institutes of Health (1985). Consensus development conference statement: Lowering blood cholesterol to prevent heart disease. *JAMA, 253,* 2080–2086.

Peterson, G.S., Lefebvre, R.C., & Ferreira, A. (1968). Strategies for cholesterol lowering at the worksite. *Journal of Nutrition Education, 18*(2), S54–S57.

Pocock, S.J., Shaper, A.G., & Phillips, A.N. (1989). Concentrations of high density lipoprotein cholesterol, triglycerides, and total cholesterol in ischemic heart disease. *The British Journal of Medicine, 72,* 998–1002.

Quigley, H.L. (1986). L.L. Bean cholesterol reduction program. *Journal of Nutrition Education, 18*(2) S58–S59.

Sempos, C., Fulwood, R., Haines, C., & Cleeman, J. (1989). The prevalence of high blood cholesterol levels among adults in the United States. *JAMA, 262,* 45–51.

Notes:

Notes:

Notes: